I0409604

10 Key Strategies
for
EASY Weight Loss

Mastering the Inner Game

Katie Darden

www.ABodyYouLove.com

Career Life Press
PO Box 282
Trinidad, CA 95570
United States of America

Copyright Notice

Copyright © 2009 - 2012 by Katie Darden.
All Rights Reserved.

Reproduction or translation of any part of this work beyond that permitted by section 107 or 108 of the 1976 United States Copyright Act without permission of the copyright owner is unlawful. Requests for permission or further information should be addressed to the author.

Katie Darden, Career Life Press
PO Box 282, Trinidad, CA, 95570,
United States of America
www.ABodyYouLove.com

This publication is designed to provide accurate and authoritative information in regard to the subject matter covered. It is sold the understanding that the author and publisher are not engaged in rendering legal, accounting, medical or other professional services. If legal, medical or other expert assistance or advice is required, the services of a competent professional should be sought. As with all self-help programs, it is the reader's responsibility to use common sense and seek appropriate medical or other professional advice before embarking on their own program. No specific results are promised or guaranteed, and the author accepts no responsibility for how the reader may choose to use or implement this information.

First Printing, 2012

ISBN-13: 978-1481983112

ISBN-10: 1481983113

Printed in the United States of America

Contents

From Here to There - And Back Again

If you're like me, you've spent far too many years trying diet after diet after diet! Some even worked – but not for long. Because diets require extraordinary efforts or wildly different eating or exercising habits, they never really get integrated into your lifestyle.

So, after the diet is "over" you go back to your regular habits – sometimes quickly, sometimes slowly, but eventually you go back to the same habits that got you into trouble in the first place!!

I first got on the roller coaster diet yo-yo back in high school and I never got off. I've tried a ton of diets and programs. I've had moderate success and varying results. Even those diets and programs that did seem to work only worked for a while - I couldn't seem to get them to stick.

Then, for over 10 years I hit one of those dieting plateaus. Nothing seemed to work at all, and in fact the weight just keep creeping up. I went back to several diets that had worked before, but this time nothing seemed to help.

Having gone through so many diets and programs, I had learned many of the "secrets" - eat less than you use, exercise regularly, etc. - but just as the "buy low, sell high" wisdom in the financial world is not so easy to implement, there still seemed to be something missing. I couldn't always get the new habits or the new eating plans to "stick". And added to that, in the past several years, nothing seemed to help to get the weight off.

Finally I decided enough was enough and set out to find something – anything – that could take me back to a weight that made me feel good, a weight I could maintain.

I discovered a program that promised results. I tried it and sure enough, with plenty of focus and work, I eventually dropped 55 pounds of fat.

I was ecstatic that something finally seemed to work for getting rid of the excess weight. And, in the process, it actually filled in a couple more missing pieces about how to get weight off and keep it off.

After only one month on the program, my husband and I went on our first cruise. By that time I had learned enough about my own body and how to eat that I actually lost 7 pounds, even while enjoying the meals and desserts onboard the ship. My coach said I was probably the only person in the history of cruising to actually lose weight on a cruise!

Life Steps In

But, then as I got closer to reaching my goal, life stepped back in and most of the weight came back. True, it took a lot longer to come back than it did for me to lose it. And not all of it came back. But enough to send me questing again.

So I set out to understand and conquer this from a strategic point of view, instead of simply anecdotal or haphazard guessing. After all, I was a Business and Career Coach who advocated a strategic approach to business planning and goal setting.

I have been successful in most areas of my life, and have accomplished nearly everything I set out to do. So this time I examined what had worked for me in the past - not just about weight, but other areas too - and figured out what I needed to shift in order to conquer this problem. If you're interested in the details of what I went through, you can read more about my personal weight story at the end of this book. There's bound to be something in there that you can identify with.

As a result of my search and the shifts I've made, I am now clear that it's an inner game. So long as I am conscious of my relationship with food, I need never have a weight problem again. It takes time and awareness, but if you are willing to commit to your own health and wellbeing, then you really can learn the pieces necessary to manage your weight successfully and unconsciously.

This book covers what I consider to be several of the key strategies leading to that success. You've probably heard of most of these strategies before. Just because the concepts I talk about seem simple doesn't necessarily mean they will be easy to understand or implement. It took me many years to figure them out, and I'm still learning.

Over the years I've discovered that in order to be successful - regardless of our focus - we need to take a holistic approach. We must include all the elements of who we are - physical, mental, emotional and even spiritual - and consider how to ensure they are all taken care of in the process. In the psychological realm, this includes what's called an ecology check. That means the decision(s) can't be evaluated in a vacuum.

A Balanced Approach

You can't adopt behaviors that benefit you in one area but jeopardize another and expect to have success - at least not for long. If you've read any of my other books, you already know I advocate a balanced (ecological) approach for most things, especially for goals.

The bottom line is I want you to be successful. I want you to get rid of the yo-yo forever. I want you to finally have a sense of control over whatever demons brought you here. I want you to recognize your value and your worth. I want you and need you as a contributing player in life.

Even though there is a spiritual aspect to this, I promise not to bring religion into it. But you are welcome to overlay any religious views you may have, especially if they are part of your support system. And I promise not to get too "new age-y" or woo-woo.

At the same time, I will be introducing you to brain and mind technology that sometimes feels like magic. I will include Neuro Linguistic Programming (NLP) and hypnosis techniques that seem to blast through mental barriers and bring rapid shifts. If you're someone who prefers to listen to an audio recording of the exercises, you'll find a link in the Resources section where you can get information about how to purchase an audio version.

I'll offer some specific techniques in each of the strategies. Some will work for you and some may not. Hopefully you'll discover new ways to apply the information, ways that fit your own unique situation.

I'll also recommend resources and provide links for information and tools that I've found useful. I'll ask you to be uncomfortable and to step outside your own paradigm to consider new things. And I will be honest about my own journey down this road.

I'm Not Perfect

So, let's be clear: I'm not perfect. As I write this I am actively using these same strategies on my own path back to healthy weight management - to losing the nearly 50 pounds that literally inched their way back onto my body.

And I'm not an expert - at least not for anyone else but myself. I don't know your situation and I wouldn't attempt to tell you what you should do. But I certainly can share what's worked for me. And I'm willing to share how and where I got stuck and unstuck. And maybe some of it will be useful for you. Make no mistake, I'm still on this journey, too.

But you know how that light bulb goes on in the instant of enlightenment? That mental snap of fingers when something becomes clear? That moment when you are so "in the flow" it feels like nothing can stop you? That's where I am right now in my journey.

I've been looking for the "answers" ever since puberty when my weight suddenly became a "problem". I've spent countless hours trying to figure out how and why it happened. I know when, and I know why, but that didn't help to reduce my weight nor keep it off.

I've even had various periods where weight was simply not an issue - some as long as four years. Periods where it seemed easy for the weight to stay off and I thought my searching might be over. That perhaps I'd never have to face extra weight and extra fat again.

But the weight always seemed to come back. Sometimes it came back suddenly, seemingly overnight (40 pounds in 3 months?). Often it came back with no apparent change in eating habits.

Finally I Get It

In a training program I took many years ago they used to say that "understanding" was the booby prize. If you "understand" a joke, you can dissect it, you can explain it, but it isn't funny. On the other hand, if you "get" a joke, there's that instant connection - you laugh, you understand - you "get" a huge pay off.

That's what this journey was about for me. I spent several decades trying to understand and figure it out, but the solution always eluded me. Until now. Because now I "get" it. Big difference involving a subtle shift.

Finally I "get" the dynamics of what happened and what that means. I know how I got off track and how to not only get back on, but also how to stay there.

This time, I'm not desperate. I'm not stuck with relying upon willpower and determination. Willpower requires being forceful, forcing something into or onto something that is resistant. It's hard to keep up willpower. It's a struggle and always results in fatigue at some point. Once you get tired or discouraged, you end up letting down, and that leads to failure. I'm through with struggle.

I am not stuck in "hope" - hoping that this new thing (diet, drug, program) will help. The problem with "hope" is that it always includes an element of failure. When you "hope" that something will be successful, you are also including the possibility of things not working out the way you wanted. I prefer to not leave that door open.

This time I'm the one in control. I understand what works (and why). I am applying what I've learned from and about these strategies in a fully conscious manner. I've integrated the strategies and techniques that were successful for me with other things in the past - like giving up cigarettes and caffeine. And I've chosen to totally eliminate the need to be perfect, since that's often the very thing that sabotages our success.

This book is written by a woman, so it (naturally) has a woman's point of view. But I am speaking to that wonderfully creative source within each of us. The part of us that wants to sing and dance and fly. That part that somehow got trapped inside this snowsuit of a body and would love to be able to simply take it off and be free again. That spark that already knows what needs to be done, but may be feeling stuck because it's forgotten how.

Everyone's Journey Is Different

I don't know where you are starting from. I don't know your personal story about how you got here. I do know that the Universe brought us together because you are reading this book. So, there must be something of value here for you. My goal is to make it easy for you to find your nugget(s), and successful in applying them.

Because this is a journey, you'll have several opportunities to engage in written exercises designed to help you identify specific components of your own challenges as well as successes. These exercises work best if you record your answers in a notebook or journal. That way you can refer back to your notes when needed.

Some people like to record everything. Some are more comfortable with statistics and others with writing out their feelings. Do whatever works for you, but be open to experimenting. And please make some kind of record - you'll be glad you did. Besides, writing things down often moves them from inside your head and frees up mental resources to find better, more resourceful solutions.

I don't advocate any particular diet or weight loss program. Different people have different results based upon their genetic, lifestyle and physical health needs. And the results can vary at different times in their lives. I've learned for myself that what worked for me 20 years ago doesn't work today.

And, I'm not a fan of fads. I'm in this for the long term. What I'm presenting here are ideas you can use with whatever diet program you want. Or, you can be like me, and decide that since this is for the rest of my life, I'm through with artificial, restrictive diets. I'm using these strategies to modify my habits and behaviors in the "real world".

Rather than artificially restricting certain foods, I'll be conscious of what I eat and when, paying attention to my body and its needs. I'll apply these strategies in a way that supports optimal health. I finally get to be a thin person.

The first strategy is rather long, but it has to be because that's where we set the foundation with a couple of very important exercises. Do yourself a favor and don't just read through the exercises. Actually do the work. You'll be glad you did.

The rest of the strategies include practical information as well as some specific exercises and processes based on the focus of that chapter. But each of these strategies are really basic common sense. I call them Easy because they are simple and relatively straightforward. But we as human beings like to complicate stuff. For some reason, we like to add lots of rules and modifiers that take things from easy to hard.

Don't read too much into these strategies, and don't over-complicate. Unless, of course, that's something you like to do. And if that's you, you might want to ask yourself what you gain from doing that and how well is it serving you?

These 10 Key Strategies are based on my own personal weight loss journey. It wouldn't be complete without my own story, so I've included it at the end of the book. Feel free to read it now if you wish, or wait until you have completed going through the Strategies. It's not an essential read, but it does provide some insight into how I discovered these strategies.

No matter how you choose to use the information in this book, I want to congratulate you on your desire to gain mastery in your own life. And to welcome you to the journey.

~Strategy 1~
Start With Yourself – Not With The Diets Out There

You are the most important person in the world. You. Yes, YOU.

Regardless of what anyone else, anywhere, could ever say or do, You are the most important person in your world. You have to be. Without You, Your Personal World, Your Personal Point of View could never exist.

So, for the sake of this conversation, and since we're talking about the very private world of You, You are the Most Important Person in the World.

I want you to keep this in mind as we go through the strategies in this book.

It doesn't matter what anyone, anywhere else thinks about what we'll be discussing here. The only one who matters is You. This is Your World, and only You will know what resonates and what will work for you. I'll share lots of ideas about what's worked for me, and I encourage you to be open to hearing new ideas, but only YOU will be able to assess the results for yourself. Not me, not your mom, not your best friend, not your Health Coach. Only You.

And it's important to clear that up right away.

If you are wanting to lose weight for someone else, because someone else thinks you should, or because you want to be attractive to some other person, it will never last. You will find yourself back on that diet yo-yo before you know it. However, if you're ready to make this transition because it's right and correct for YOU, then you've just given your chances for success an exponential boost. Welcome Aboard!

Make no mistake - this is a journey of incredible selfishness and focus. It couldn't be any other way. You can't live your life for anyone else, just as no one else can live for you. The choices that you make must be for you, and you alone. If other people get some kind of enjoyment or benefit from it, fine. But to have any chance for success, this has to be for you, and you alone, no matter how selfish that may sound.

You are unique. Your point of view is unique. Your body is unique. Your gifts and talents are unique. Your approach to life is unique. Your lifestyle is unique. This is a wonderful thing. The world needs each and every one of us, playing full out, at the top of our game. The contribution you have to make in the world is not like anyone else's, and given the condition of the world today, we need your creative contributions more than ever.

However, in order to make a contribution, you need to be Here, in the Physical World. And to be here long enough to share your gifts, you need to be healthy.

If you are struggling with your weight, then there is some kind of conflict going on for you that is interfering with your natural birthright. Our purpose here is to eliminate that conflict so you can get on with making the contribution you came here to make.

The most important thing you can do in any weight control, weight loss, or weight maintenance program is to remember that You Are Unique and so your plan must also be unique to you and your needs. Your plan must fit not only your body type, it must also fit your personality, your lifestyle and your preferences. Otherwise, it's bound to fail and you are bound to feel like a failure. And that's counterproductive to making a contribution to the world.

The importance of understanding your personal uniqueness is why diets, even when they have initial success, ultimately are difficult to maintain. Most diets have mandatory "rules" that interfere with our natural inclinations, our chosen lifestyles and our normal eating habits.

Anything that takes effort will be difficult to maintain. If you're reading this book then I have to assume you want your weight loss to be permanent. You want your efforts to mean something that is sustainable. ***But not at the expense of being yourself.***

How Will You Know You Are Successful?

I want you to take some time, right now, to think about what it will take for you to feel successful in your healthy weight goals. What will you need (to be, achieve, acquire, let go of) in order to consider yourself successful? This is (or should be) about the rest of your life. You'll want to set yourself up to be successful right from the start. So take the time right now to figure out how that success would look and feel once you've achieved it. How would you know?

This is a good time to record your thoughts and ideas in your journal. Write it down, look it over. Modify as necessary. Make it real.

The next thing to consider is WHY you want it. Make this very personal. Not for anyone else but you. When you articulate your "compelling why", you'll actually begin the process of commitment, the process of owning your dreams. Again, write your notes in your journal.

Spend whatever time is necessary to create a full, rich, descriptive picture for yourself.

Throughout the rest of this book we'll explore some individual strategies and techniques to help you attain your goal. But we have to start at the beginning.

So, as we've already discussed, to begin with, you must recognize that the choice to be healthy has to start with YOU. Like any other major life change, it must be about YOU and for YOU. Not for anyone else.

When you recognize you're ready and actually make the commitment for health, these strategies will seem easy to implement. It won't take will-power or any special tools or foods to be successful. It **will** take acknowledging that you are worth it, along with choosing to adopt new habits. And, it will take your commitment to see your choices through to reaching your inevitable success.

Where Our Beliefs Come From

In order to have the success you want, you must first recognize your own natural worth. You *do* recognize that you're worthy, don't you?

Unfortunately, many of us grow up in families or situations where we adopt the idea on some subtle level that we are **not** worthy. This is true across the board, not just for those who are born into a specific financial or cultural strata, and not just for those of us who have weight issues.

Most beliefs start when we're young, often before we're five years old. During those formative years we're little sponges, soaking up what's told to us, what we observe, and paying close attention to the wishes of our parents or other authority figures.

We believe and trust the adults around us, often unconsciously absorbing their beliefs as our own. We listen to what they say, assuming it to be true. We interpret, in our own limited way, what their actions mean about and toward us. We learn what it feels like to feel "bad" and we decide not to feel that way, so we modify our behavior in ways we believe will avoid that feeling.

We want the love and approval of the adults around us, and we are dependent upon them for our very survival. Unfortunately we haven't yet developed the critical thinking that helps us determine what's true and what's not.

Most of the influential adults in our early lives were simply doing the best they could to raise and protect us, even when what they were attempting to do was misguided or mistaken.

They may have criticized or cautioned us, believing that they were helping us, when in fact, without knowing it, their words or actions were crippling us. Sometimes it happened through implication and sometimes it was intentional, but often it was simply the result of our own interpretation of a comment from someone else.

It didn't even have to be real. If it was simply your interpretation, that made it real enough for you to believe that it was true.

So in our young, naive way, we took to heart what these people we respected (or feared) said to us, often adopting their point of view, and generally believing that their perception defined us. And in our desire to please them, to get along, or to respect their "authority" (unless we were totally rebellious), we often allowed their belief to throw doubt on or overshadow our own when there was conflict.

Even worse, some of us tried to be "perfect" as a way to gain their acceptance or approval. Often the attempt for perfection is our own desire to feel like we fit in or belong, an attempt to overcorrect for our deep-seated sense of unworthiness.

Our Conscious and Unconscious Minds

Most of this happens below the level of full conscious awareness. The subconscious (or unconscious) mind is always at work. It's tasked with keeping us alive, so it's where the functioning of the autonomic nervous system is regulated - it keeps you breathing, your heart beating, your cells working properly, etc.

As a result of my own research and observations, I believe the unconscious part of our mind is also where most of our emotional reactions originate. I think that our emotions are our lightening-fast reactions to the world around us. The unconscious is tasked with keeping us healthy and alive. So where animals have instincts, we humans have emotions.

When something happens, our unconscious mind reads the cues very quickly and lets loose with emotions that give us clues to survival. We become afraid, we laugh, we feel an instant attraction to someone else.

The unconscious has been working for us ever since birth. That means that some of the reactions, responses, or habits originated at a time long before we had the ability to create rational decisions for ourselves. We made incomplete interpretations based on what we "knew" at the time.

I have a conscious memory of sitting on a porch step at 5 years of age, having seen a movie about unrequited love and thinking wistfully, "that's just the way life is." Now seriously, what does a 5 year old know about adult love?

But that's what happened to many of us - we interpreted the events around us and made decisions at an early age, and we continue to act and react to life as if those early beliefs were true, never questioning and often never even aware of where the decisions or judgments came from in the first place. Think about it - would you allow a 5 year old to tell you how to run your life? Well, in many ways, that's exactly what you're doing.

Luckily, the unconscious mind can be negotiated with. When we become aware of behaviors that no longer support us, we can often modify the behaviors so that they actually are based on what is in our own best interests. The unconscious mind's role is to protect us and our sense of who we are. So how we "see" ourselves is vitally important.

Recognizing Your Worth

In my opinion, lack of self-worth (which shows up as lack of self-confidence or lack of self-esteem) is probably the number one issue facing people today. This serious problem stops us from achieving our goals because it causes us to believe we don't **deserve** to have success.

This is so important that it's one of the very first things we need to address. Otherwise, no matter what you attempt, you will never give yourself full permission to be successful.

So, let's get over that one right now.

We'll be engaging our conscious and unconscious minds in several different processes throughout the rest of the book. As we work with the conscious mind you'll be recording things you observe. When we work with the unconscious mind you will focusing more on internal pictures, representations and in some cases, sensations. Rapid changes usually happen on the unconscious level and then get relayed to conscious awareness where we can notice more of the subtleties and nuances of what's going on.

Without going into too many details, the conscious mind is where you "let things stew" when you want to mull things over. That little flash of insight you sometimes get? It's the unconscious relaying information to you after it's been processed.

Letting Go of False Beliefs

First, we'll start by engaging our rational conscious mind to focus our attention. Then we'll engage our unconscious mind to support us in shifting our internal representations.

Take a few moments to think about the people in your life who you think have made you feel unworthy in some way. If you get stuck, just think about how you feel when you're with other people, and identify the ones who make you feel like you're not quite as good as they are.

Remember, they may not have done anything on purpose. In fact, they may not have done anything at all. Because of the way our minds work, it could all be imaginary. But that doesn't make it any less "real" in terms of how it affects you.

In your journal, make a list of the individuals, draw a line down the page and next to their names, write a brief description of what they said, what they did, or what it was that made you feel not quite good enough.

When you look at your list, ask yourself if their perception about or their action towards you was accurate. I'm willing to bet that in at least 90% of the cases their thinking was flawed. Perhaps they didn't know you, didn't understand you, or had their own selfish interests at heart.

But this isn't about them. It's about YOU. You can't change them, even if what they did was on purpose. But you **can** change you. You can change your reaction to the situation. You can change your perception of the situation. And if you believed them, even just a little, you can change that, too. All it takes is willingness, commitment, and a little bit of work.

So look at your list, going down it line by line. Look at each person and circumstance, and ask yourself if it is, or was, true. Not whether that person believed it was true, but was **their** perception about **you** (or the circumstance) true.

As you get to each perception or circumstance, cross out the ones that you know are not true, or that no longer apply. Do this for the entire list.

Now go back through your list, this time looking at each person. Recognize that the person is human, and just as flawed as you or anyone else. That means, that at the time the incident happened, they were doing the best they could with what they had. You were simply an actor in their play, and while their words or actions may have seemed personal to you, *their play is about them*. Their actions and reactions were about **them**. Not about you, even if you may have contributed to what happened.

As you go through the list this time, remind yourself that you may have been the *target*, but you were (probably) not the *cause* of what they were personally going through at that moment. And if you were the cause, then perhaps you have some additional cleaning up to do yourself. Ask yourself if you are ready to forgive that person for the way they treated you, or the way they thought about you. Then cross out each person's name as you forgive them.

There may be one or two people on your list that are hard for you to forgive. The person may have been very important to your survival as a child (like a parent or teacher). They may have imposed great harm on you. You may still feel some kind of pain as a result of your interaction with them.

However, remember, *you* are the one feeling the pain, not *them*. And ask yourself if it's worthwhile for you to carry that pain or anger around. A friend of mine refers to this as "letting someone else live rent free in your head". You'd never let someone live rent free in your house, why would you let them live rent free in your head?

Chances are that the anger or pain you are carrying, or the need to protect yourself from it, has become part of the insulation on your body that we commonly called fat.

So now you get to choose, forgiveness or pain? Forgiveness or Fat?

Then go back through the list of remaining names, and ask yourself for each one, what will it take for you to be willing to let go of your anger or pain and forgive that person? And, are you willing to let go of it, in order to have what you really want?

It may be useful here for you to remember that forgiving does not mean you have to forget. The pain you have felt is real. Pain is always a warning signal, it's there in order to get your attention. But that doesn't mean that you have to believe the person, the words, or the perception that caused the pain.

In fact, in most cases, the pain you feel is because you know that person's perception (or your interpretation of it) is **not** accurate. It feels painful because if it **were** true, it would mean that you are in opposition to (and disconnected from) your true self (and your true worth).

At the heart of everything, in that place where you are connected to the source of all being (however you chose to think of it - God, Universe, Higher Self), you know the truth of who you are. And no one can touch that.

So it feels painful when you consider that someone else's mistaken perception may be true. In other words, you may feel bad when something makes you feel unworthy. The pain or unease is not because you **are** unworthy, it's because when you think of being unworthy you know at your core it isn't true. It's a warning signal to you that your thinking at that moment is screwy and that adopting it will cause the disconnection that you are worried about. When we pay attention to these signals, they are alerting us to where our thinking is off track. You never have to believe anyone else's perception of you.

Let's face it, if you **were** unworthy, it would just be a "so what". It would be a fact of life like having brown hair or big ears. And that fact wouldn't cause you as much grief or pain as being called something that isn't true.

If you need some additional help to forgive some of the people on your list, here's an adaptation of Steve Andreas' forgiveness technique that may make it easier for you. It's a process that will allow you to let go of your upset. It does not require you to forget anything that happened to you. It simply assists you in shifting your feelings about what happened, which in turn frees you to move on.

You'll get much more benefit when you take the time to actually go through these steps, not just read it to get to the rest of the information in the book.

Some people find it easier to listen to someone talk them through these kinds of processes. If that's you, I've included a link in the Resources section where you can purchase an audio version of the exercises in this book.

Alternatively, you can record this into a digital format and listen to it. But you can also simply read through the italicized instructions and then mentally walk yourself through the steps.

The Forgiveness Process

Set aside 15-20 minutes. Find a place to sit and relax with no interruptions. Read through these instructions, and then close your eyes and take yourself through the process. Or, simply listen to the recording that I (or you) created.

Close your eyes and take a deep breath. Imagine you have a large blank screen in front of you that extends slightly beyond the edges of your vision. Sort of like a movie screen in the theatre, but this one is 3-dimensional so there is also depth to it.

Now think about someone you have already forgiven, someone you have known for a while. This should be someone whose actions or words caused enough pain that you felt angry or upset, in some way estranged from them. Then at some point you forgave them. You released your pain and you no longer feel any upset with or around them. Preferably, this should be someone who is still in your life.

Imagine that person in the space in front of you. When you think about them, having already forgiven them, notice where they are located on your screen. Pay attention to the details you notice about them. For instance, when I think of people I've forgiven, they are always located in the upper right, off in the distance a bit, slightly above eye level.

Once you've identified your own "forgiven" location, think about someone from your list that you have not yet been able to forgive, but that you now want to.

When you think about that not-yet-forgiven person, notice the location on your screen where they show up. For me, those people tend to be slightly to my left, at eye level, and closer in towards me.

Take a moment to notice all the differences between these two people you are imagining - the location, the size, the relative closeness or distance, the brightness or dimness, the clarity or fuzziness of the image. Is there a physical sensation for you? Are there sounds associated with either or both representations? Noises or words?

These details are part of your internal representation system. They are called "submodalities" and are clues to how your brain codes your experience. In this case it's the experience of forgiveness.

In other words, you are discovering how your brain recognizes that you have forgiven someone.

Once you have noted all the differences (and it's sometimes useful to write them down for future reference), focus on your internal representation of the person you want to forgive but have so far been unable to.

Now start applying the submodalities you identified for the forgiven to the unforgiven person. This is called "mapping". You want to make the submodalities for the unforgiven person as similar to the forgiven as you can.

Once that's done, move your image of the unforgiven person into the same spatial location as the forgiven.

If you are like most people, you will feel an immediate shift in how you think of that person who was previously unforgiven. Many people report a sense of ease or relaxation, a lessening of tension, or a wash of love.

Sometimes the previously unforgiven person doesn't seem to want to stay in the forgiven location. That just means that you are not yet ready to forgive them. You can ask yourself mentally what it will take for you to be willing to forgive that person.

Pay attention to the information you get, but remember - this is about YOU, not about them. If you are requiring them to do or be something, then it may be a very long time before you have closure.

If you discovered something new, go back through the process again and map across any new information you may have noticed. Then move the person again into the forgiven location.

If they still don't stick, or "feel" right, ask yourself what it will take for you to be willing to forgive them.

Now that you have identified your submodalities regarding forgiveness, you will be able to move through this process relatively easily. In fact, if you have several similar unforgiven people on your list, you might try doing a "batch" forgiveness to take care of several all at once.

Once you have forgiven all of the people on your list, or all of those that you can at this time, congratulate yourself on a job well done and open your eyes.

While reading through these processes is useful, to get the full value, make sure you actually go back and do the exercise as it's written.

Now, line through the rest of the people on your list who are now forgiven. The next time you realize you need to forgive someone, you now have the tools to take care of it quickly.

Once you're through with that step, there's one more task that you must complete.

This time, make a list of all of the major areas where you have claimed to yourself that you are not worthy. This will be a list of those things where you feel (or have felt) inferiority, shame, guilt, or even remorse. This might be a very long list if you take the time to look at every specific instance.

But we don't need a full laundry list of everything - this is not meant to be a confessional. Besides we want to get on with our lives, and dwelling on this kind of thing doesn't serve to move us forward, it keeps us stuck in the past. That's the opposite of what we want. What you can do instead, is to think of general categories, and use one or two examples to describe each.

Next, go down the list of areas or circumstances and ask yourself if it is really true that you are not worthy in that area. Cross off all of the perceptions, circumstances or areas that you know to be false. In some cases you'll discover you've been thinking of yourself as "not good enough" when in reality it might simply be that you don't know enough - yet. That's not a major character flaw - it's something that's fixable.

When you have completed this activity, take a few moments to ask yourself if you are willing to forgive **yourself** for having been so judgmental as to assume that you are anything less than the perfect you. This doesn't mean that you don't have faults, or that you will always do everything exactly the way that it is supposed to be done.

What being the "perfect you" means, is that given who you are at this moment, what you know and what you have available to you, you are being the best and doing the best that you can.

And, in truth, that is always the case. But it's easy for us to forget it, especially if we compare ourselves to others. Or, when we set an impossible standard for ourselves. In those cases we are simply setting ourselves up for failure.

When you are consciously identifying your values, there are some specific ways you must think about them. And, you need to create standards that eliminate the potential for self-sabotage and make sure you can "win". In my **Core Values** book we focus on how to identify what's most important to you and how to create your personal "rules" that ensure you will be successful. Most of us set unrealistic expectations of ourselves.

I'm not advocating that you use excuses to avoid taking responsibility. I'm simply saying that each of us does the best that we can, with what we have at the moment. There is always room for improvement, and there's always room for growth. If we focus on finding fault with ourselves, we limit our ability to discover and to implement that improvement.

That's why your health and weight journey has to be for *you*, not for anyone else. The sooner you learn to accept who you are, to recognize and believe in your own (spiritual) connection to your best self, and to love yourself for the gifts you have to contribute to this world, the sooner you can be successful in your journey. And the sooner the rest of us will get to celebrate you in our own lives.

Reconnecting With Your Source

So now, it's time to forgive yourself for being shortsighted or for believing what someone else may have thought or implied about you, even if they were a parent, teacher or other "authority". And for accepting the idea that what they said or did had anything to do with you.

In the next exercise we'll take the opportunity to reconnect to our own inner sense of what is right and just, and make a commitment to trust our own best judgment from now on.

Give yourself 10-15 minutes. Again, you may want to read through it first and then do the process yourself. If you have the audio version, you can read first, or just go ahead and listen.

Take a deep breath and close your eyes. Take another deep breath and as you release it, let yourself relax even more.

Think of a favorite place you like to go, or one where you used to go as a child. Imagine yourself there now. This does not have to be a real place.

Imagine you are watching a younger version of yourself in this location. Watch yourself playing and observing the things around you. Hear the sounds of the location and simply enjoy how it feels to be there.

Remember what it felt like to be fully immersed in just being. No worries, no concerns, no doubts, no pressure. Free to just relax and enjoy the moment.

Relax even more into the moment, drinking in all the enjoyment of your surroundings. As you watch this younger version of yourself, recognize the inherent goodness this young being represents. Notice the glow of life, the relative innocence, the rightness of being.

As you observe this being, imagine a beam of golden light that flows down from the sky, bathing this younger you in warm radiant life-giving light, connecting you to the Universe and all that is healthy and whole, all that is good and god-like.

Imagine this younger you looks up and into your eyes, a smile forming. This younger you, still glowing, walks over to where you are standing, and smiling, takes your hand.

You feel the instant connection, the recognition, remembering who you are and have always been at the core of your being.

You hug this younger you in a warm embrace and notice that the glowing light flows into your body too, permeating and awakening the healthy life force in all of your cells, creating a sort of glowing halo surrounding and protecting your body.

You are once again reconnected, to your own Higher Self, the Universe, and all that is good. You remember what it feels like to trust yourself, even if the last time was long, long ago. And you know, now, that you can come back here anytime you need to refresh.

As you release your younger you, you watch as the child slips away into the surrounding area, waving playfully.

You stand for a moment, basking in the glow that still surrounds you, the connection to all-that-is, understanding that you belong here just as the trees, birds, flowers and all of life. You have much to contribute and much to share. You realize your body is just the vehicle, your means for moving through the world. It is a useful thing, this body and it's here to help you, to keep you connected to the physical realm.

You are always connected to your spirit, and your spirit is always connected to the larger Universe... and so you can let go of the worries and stress of living in a physical body in the physical world. You can release yourself from the mistaken beliefs that have held you back from sharing your innermost gifts. You are free to return to the physical world and be your true self, knowing you are connected to your spirit which is there to assist and guide you.

As you stand basking in the glow that still envelops you, you can begin to feel yourself releasing more and more of any remaining stress, worry, hesitation or tension.

You let it flow back to the Universe, out through your glowing cells, letting it intermingle with the other atoms and molecules, to be transformed into something even more useful.

You notice the glow around you begins to subside, condensing into a small warm ball that gives off a glow like an ember centered in the region of your heart, and you realize this is the connection that is always there, always ready to be called forward again when needed.

The calming glow is the center of your creativity, health and loving spirit as made manifest by your physical body here on earth.

Take a deep breath in, and enjoy the calmness and connection.

When you are fully relaxed and ready to get on with your day, go ahead and open your eyes, remembering that you can return to this inner space and calm anytime you wish.

Aligning With Your Body and Health Goals

The next step in the process of gaining control over your health and well-being as it relates to your physical body, is to identify your specific goals, and move yourself into alignment with them. You won't have true success until you can do that. Once you recognize that you deserve to have the body and lifestyle you want, it will be easy to maintain the healthy choices.

So consider the questions in the list below. Think about the kinds of things you already know about yourself and what you will need to take into consideration when adopting and adapting the upcoming strategies:

- Am I willing to make myself **#1** in terms of my eating and health?
- Am I willing to keep moving forward and quickly get back on track if I deviate?
- Am I willing to make lifestyle changes in order to sustain my progress?
- Am I willing to keep myself accountable for the commitment I've made?
- Specifically, what issues in my life, lifestyle or work must I take into consideration in order to make this successful? (You may want to write these out since you will need to develop your own personal strategies to keep them aligned with your new commitment.

Take a moment to define **exactly** what you are committed to. Make it health-oriented versus weight- or size-oriented. In other words, while focusing on a particular weight can be useful as a long term end-goal, you want to set yourself up to be, and to remain, successful.

For instance, it's easier to be successful when you commit to not eating starches than it is to losing five pounds in a week. Your goal may be the five pounds, but you may not have control over your metabolism, your cortisol, your water-retention. You do have control over what you put in your mouth.

Also, make it simple and easy for yourself. Remember that many diet plans fail because they are so complex and have too many rigid rules. Use common sense - the things you already know about yourself, your body and your lifestyle. Be reasonable, but firm.

You must be able to see yourself having the results you want. If you can't imagine actually having those results, then you will sabotage yourself. This is why we did the earlier exercises. It was important to release any pre-conceptions or limitations that would prevent us from being able to have what we want and deserve. Feel free to go back and use these exercises whenever you want or need.

Write down your commitment(s) and look at your list every morning when you get up, every night before sleep, and remind yourself of the items often during the day (before meals if that helps, too). If you have a picture of yourself looking the way you want to (AND it doesn't make you feel negative or unsuccessful - in other words it's a positive reinforcement), that can also be a great way to remind yourself of your goals. Posting your written or visual commitment on your refrigerator or bathroom mirror might be the perfect place for a reminder.

How do you know your optimum size or weight? Again, that will be individual to you and your lifestyle. While doctors have weight charts based on gender, age, body structure, etc., only you know what is best for you. While I have actually been at the "optimal" weight based on the doctor's chart, I always felt healthier when I was about 10 pounds heavier than what the chart indicated.

Remember, you don't have to be perfect – in fact, perfect is often the saboteur when it comes to sustaining any change. Instead, be committed to getting back on track if and when the need arises, and to being connected to the "perfect you".

Diets are simply tools to get you started. Most of them were never meant to be a full-time lifestyle choice. Feel free to use a diet if it helps kickstart your commitment. But remember, we are looking for lifetime sustainable health, not just a short-term aid.

Congratulate yourself for every small win - and forgive yourself when you transgress, but get back on the bandwagon immediately if you make a mistake.

Once you've completed these very important first steps in this chapter, we'll shift gears and look at some specific strategies that will help support you in achieving your new lifestyle goals...

~Strategy 2~
Less IS More

How and when you eat can make as much of a difference as *what* you eat.

Eating small portions every 2-1/2 to 3 hours, rather than the often "recommended" 3 square meals a day can go a long way to ensuring your success in shifting your eating habits to meet your health goals.

You've probably heard that people who "graze" are generally less likely to have issues with their weight.

That's because they pay attention to when and how their body demands food. They never get too hungry, which means they are less likely to be tempted by foods that are not nutritionally sound. In other words, they're not going after fast food and donuts – food that may taste yummy but has little or no nutritional value for the body.

Most people actually wait too long between their meals. By limiting your meals to only three times a day, you are generally going to be more hungry when lunch or dinner time comes, and you will overeat because of that hunger. Anything you overeat becomes fat that gets stored on the body to take care of those times when you are hungry and can't eat. This starts that cycle of "feast or famine" and causes the body to hold on to the fat stores as if they are precious.

Recent studies have shown that it's actually the total daily caloric intake that counts, regardless of how you spread it across the day. So it apparently doesn't matter a whole lot (calorie-wise) if you eat everything at one sitting, or split it into 6 smaller meals.

The problem with "3 square meals a day" – at least for those of us with a weight issue – is that when we arbitrarily have a set number of meals, or if we deny ourselves a healthy snack when we're hungry, we're a lot more likely to overeat at our next meal. And that, in turn, sets up the expectation that all our meals should be large ones.

When you eat smaller portions more frequently, or have healthy snacks between your meals, you help to control your hunger as well as your blood sugar, and you are less likely to overeat when you do sit down to a meal. By eating more frequently, you turn off your insulin pump and the cravings stop. And even better, when you eat more often you will be giving your body the energy it needs to cope throughout the day.

Have you ever watched the way a healthy child eats? One who hasn't been badgered about what and how to eat? They eat when they're hungry. That often includes a snack when they get home from school. Not a full blown meal, a small snack to tide them over.

Keeping your snacks to about 100 calories will satisfy your hunger and give your body the boost it needs, without triggering a desire to binge.

If you're wondering what (or even when) to snack, use this idea: Just as a time management guru might remind you to ask yourself, "is this the best and most useful way to spend my time at this moment?", when you are tempted to eat something outside of your normal snacks or meals, ask yourself, "is this the best and most beneficial (healthy) snack I have available at this moment?'

Checking in with yourself and then paying attention to what your *body* says (**not your mind**) is very helpful. You will often notice your body has a physical reaction when you think of a particular food. Your mind, on the other hand has an emotional reaction first (Chocolate? Did you say chocolate?) that then leads to a remembered feeling. Unfortunately the feeling is often an emotional reaction to pain or pleasure related to the food, not to the way the food affects your body.

If you're not sure whether it's your mind or your body reacting to the thought of the food, go ahead and eat it. Then take note of how you feel a couple of hours later. It might taste yummy when you eat it, but if you feel yucky later, then it's an emotionally satisfying food, not a nutritionally satisfying food.

That brings us to an important distinction. If you are making these changes a permanent part of your life, then I encourage you to only eat what you love. Forget about anything else. Even though I'm going to encourage you to eat in a way that supports your body, don't force yourself to eat anything that doesn't just sound yummy to you.

You will find, over time, that as you get back in touch with your body, it will communicate what it wants. For instance, I love broccoli, but I usually eat it just at dinner. Lately I've found that I look forward to the days when we have some leftovers because then I get to use it in my omelet the next morning. My husband on the other hand wouldn't touch that omelet with a 10 foot pole. But then, the idea of sausage (which he loves) makes me gag. One person's yum is another person's yuck.

If you have a desire for something sweet, try to substitute fresh fruit for cookies or candy. And make it whole fruit, not dried or processed, and preferably not concentrated fruit juice. By eating the whole fruit, you'll get your sugar, but you'll also get the additional nutrients that simply aren't available in processed juices and snack foods. That way your sweet tooth is taken care of and so is your body.

I know I said I wouldn't tell you what to eat, but I highly recommend you stay away from artificial sweeteners, including diet sodas. Not only are researchers finding that artificial sweeteners cause severe health problems, for those of us with weight issues, there's something even worse. The artificially sweetener bypasses our normal "shut off" switch. It simply doesn't satisfy the desire that we have for something sweet, and some people in the industry say it makes the desire or craving even worse. If you are someone who uses artificial sweeteners, I encourage you to do your own research and make up your mind.

The bottom line is that it's better for you, in the long run, to actually eat some of whatever you are craving than it is to try to avoid it. Sometimes you can substitute a healthier snack, but if it's a true craving, you just may need to give in. Pay attention to the amount, and listen to your body in an hour or so to see if you may need to do something different next time.

One of my friends was successful in losing weight precisely because she paid attention to her cravings. She permitted herself one Hershey's kiss every day as a reward for being diligent and focused. That way she never felt deprived as she made the other healthy choices during the day.

This is not an excuse to pig out on chocolate (or anything else). It's a way to pay attention and still reward yourself.

By eating smaller, nutritionally balanced meals, your body learns that it doesn't need to store calories (as fat) any longer, and in fact it can begin to burn the excess fat it has stored.

It's useful to become conscious of the amount of food you put on your plate at mealtime. If you're used to piling on 2 or 3 spoonfuls of mashed potatoes, try going for just one to begin. You can always go back for more, and when you do, you get to consider if you really want it. It becomes a conscious choice.

If you're wondering what is an "appropriate" portion, here's a useful guide. Make a fist with your hand. Look closely. That's the approximate size of your stomach at rest. That's about how much food should be on your plate. It's true that unless you've had surgery, your stomach will expand, but do you really want to be stuffed and uncomfortable? The next time you portion out your food, look at your fist.

Taking smaller portions may make you feel like you are depriving yourself at first, especially if you are used to having a certain amount of food on your plate. Some people have reported great success in using smaller plates when they eat. That way the smaller portion seems proportionate to the size of the plate.

And finally, regardless of what Mom told you, you do NOT need to clean your plate. It doesn't help the starving children anywhere when you eat every morsel because that's what you were taught. If you are still tied to that idea, then definitely make sure your portions are smaller.

However, consider this: leaving a little food on your plate may be a healthy way to remind yourself that there is enough food in the world and you do not have to worry about where your next meal is coming from. Unless you do have to worry about that, and in that case I doubt that you would be reading this book.

Think of the last time you went to a buffet. If you put something on your plate that you found you didn't like, you would never force yourself to eat all of it. Think of your meals in the same way. In a later chapter I'll talk about how to gauge your fullness and satisfaction levels. Bottom line, once your hunger is satisfied, just stop eating.

In this chapter I've talked about the importance to fueling your body on a regular basis by eating several small meals whenever you are hungry, rather that having fewer large meals or starving yourself.

The strategy discussed in this chapter is the opposite of fasting to lose weight. I'm not suggesting that intermittent fasting doesn't work for weight loss, or that fasting can't be done in a healthy way. There are too many studies that show the benefits. What we're aiming for here with the small, frequent meals, is to get away from the "feast or famine" mental and physical triggers that cause us to overeat in the first place.

If you do decide to try fasting for health reasons, be sure to read up on how to do so in a healthy manner. Like any drastic change, transitioning back is very important, so pay attention how you break your fast.

And that leads us to the next strategy ...

~Strategy 3~
Breakfast - The
Healthy Way

You've heard it before – the most important meal of the day is breakfast. That's because your body has been fasting all night while you've been sleeping. Once you awaken, you are moving out of the fasting mode and need to give your body adequate and appropriate nutritional energy to meet the demands of the day.

Even in the morning you need a balanced meal - and a Danish and coffee isn't going to hit the mark! You might think it's better than nothing, but that kind of "breakfast" is nothing but empty calories that really don't support your body and lead to other problems such as fuzzy thinking and cravings.

Your first meal of the day is important because it sets up your body and even your metabolism for the rest of the day. When you load up on sweets and sugars first thing, you set yourself up to have cravings for carbohydrates for the rest of the day. And eating simple carbohydrates is the opposite of what we want to do. As with every other meal, make sure you're getting the proper balance of protein, complex carbohydrates and healthy fat in the morning.

What "tastes good" is not always a good indicator of what your body needs. There are many online assessments you can take which will help you understand the balance that's best for your body.

I've provided a link in the Resources section to a couple of assessments from Dr. Mercola, a doctor who focuses on a nutritional approach to health. Not only does he have great articles and videos about health in general, his site has a free body-type assessment that will give you some specific information to help you understand the balance of foods that is best for your particular needs.

Each person is different, with different nutritional needs. I once tried a vegan diet where I ate nothing but fruit in the morning. I found that it was way too much sugar for me. I had a hard time focusing before lunch and I ended up gaining a bunch of weight.

That experience led me back to my earlier successes and I realized once and for all that I'm a protein gal. If you're like me and need extra protein in the morning, eggs are a great idea. Eggs are full of essential nutrients, such as vitamins A, D and E; protein; as well as choline and folate which are great for the brain and may help maintain memory as you age.

You can also add nuts to your oatmeal (especially almonds or walnuts), spread natural peanut butter on your wholegrain toast, or if you're a vegetarian, eat tofu or vegetarian sausages to make sure you get enough protein.

Regardless of what you eat in the morning, avoid refined carbohydrates (such as pastries and most commercial cereals). They are high in sugars, which unfortunately lead to the dreaded sugar crash a couple of hours later. If you've been eating cereal in the mornings (especially sugared cereals), you may have already noticed that a couple of hours later you need coffee or something else to keep you going until lunch time.

If you are using an intermittent fasting approach (where you fast for an extended period of time on a regular basis), you may want to push out your breakfast time until 10 a.m. or even noon. That way you are extending your natural overnight fasting period to get a larger benefit. Remember, though, the key here is to create a lifestyle where you don't need to go to any extremes, and as useful as fasting can be for both weight loss and health, it is an extreme.

For that reason, and especially once you get to a maintenance mode, it's best to eat breakfast within a half-hour of awakening to help set your metabolism for the day. If you never wait more than an hour after getting up in the morning before you break your fast, you are less likely to succumb to that "starved" feeling that causes you to overeat or to grab unhealthy alternatives.

Which brings us to learning how to know how much is enough ...

~Strategy 4~
Stop Eating When You Are Satisfied

Most of us live a busy, hectic lifestyle with little time for ourselves. Many of us have even forgotten what it's like to relax and enjoy our meals. Too many of us eat in our cars, standing at the kitchen counter, or sitting in front of the TV. When we eat on the run, we often have other things on our minds, and pay little attention to the food we're putting into our mouths and bodies.

An obvious first start is to pay attention to what you eat. That means to take the time to notice the food, the presentation and the tastes. Sitting down to a meal instead of grabbing something on the go will help you focus on these fundamentals. When you are distracted and not paying attention to your meal, it's much easier to overeat.

While I am not a religious person, I would like to suggest that you take a moment to give thanks anytime that you eat - even for a snack. It gives you the opportunity to slow down and be grateful for what you have. Then you can be more focused on the experience of enjoying your food and recognize when you are satisfied rather than distracted by other things.

Another key is to only eat when you're hungry. That might sound obvious, but it's amazing how many people I know who do what I call "preventative eating." They eat because they know they'll be too busy to eat later. They grab something at McDonald's or some other fast food drive through because they're going to be late for dinner.

The problem is, they are usually already hungry, so they eat something to satisfy that hunger - something that is a meal in itself - and then later they proceed to eat a full meal anyway - because it's expected that they'll eat a "normal" lunch or dinner.

If you find yourself in a situation where you need something to tide you over until your meal, make it a healthy snack. A piece of fruit, some celery or cheese. Something that takes the edge off but doesn't fill you up. If you give in and eat the equivalent of a meal, then snack later instead of doubling up.

This is one of the reasons I can't eat appetizers. When I eat them, it slakes my hunger. Then I'm not hungry enough to eat a full meal. So, unless there are enough appetizers for them to become my dinner, I simply stay away from them. The same thing is true for me with salads. I never eat my salad first. I always eat it with my meal, unless of course it IS my meal.

And then I have the girlfriend who never eats her entrée when she goes out. She eats the appetizer, the bread the salad and the dessert. And she takes the main meal to go and it becomes dinner on another night. Her thinking is that since she seldom goes out, and never eats that way at home, it's a special treat and she indulges in all the extras that she never gets. By taking the entrée home, she avoids the overeating.

How to Gauge Your Hunger Level

So how do you know when you are hungry? The first step is to be conscious of your body. For most of us with weight issues, that's easier said than done. One way is to use a mental gauge, similar to a fuel gauge in your car. Judy Wardell, in her excellent book, **Thin Within**, suggests using a Hunger Scale.

The idea is simple. Imagine you have an internal scale or gauge that reflects your hunger. The scale is calibrated from 1 to 10. When you are at 0 or 1, you are on empty. When you are at 10, you are full - stuffed like at a big Thanksgiving dinner full. When you are at 5, you are satisfied.

This makes it very simple to check in with yourself. All you do is take a moment, close your eyes, take a deep breath and relax. You can place your hand on your abdomen if you wish, it may better connect you with your bodily senses. As you sit or stand there in silence, simply ask yourself, am I feeling hungry? Where am I on my hunger scale?

If you are between 0-4, then you will be experiencing some kind of hunger. If you are between 5-10, then you are not hungry. Judy suggests that you only eat when you are below 5 and that you stop when you hit 5. That means you will continue to check in as you are eating. If you are like most overweight people, you eat to 7 or 9. Stopping at 5 insures that your body is taken care of and you are not overeating. Eating slowly is important because the stomach doesn't immediately notify the brain when it's full.

I first read about the Hunger Gauge when I read her book in the mid 1980s, and it still gives me an accurate check-in - **when I remember to use it**.

And that's an important key: *Remembering to use our effective tools until they become second nature to us.* This is called "conditioning". It is a process used by athletes and all high-performing individuals regardless of their field. Tony Robbins talks about this in all of his trainings. If you want something to become second nature, you must condition yourself until it becomes a habit.

(Important Note: when I checked on Amazon, Judy is now married and the newer versions of her book have a distinctly religious focus - a lot has happened since 1985! I have not read the new book, and I don't know how strong the religious aspect is in her new versions. I can vouch for the content in the originals, but not for whatever may have been changed.)

When it comes to hunger, there are lots of reasons why we might **think** we're hungry when in fact we're not. The most frequent reason for eating when we're not hungry is when we feel empty because of emotional reasons.

Everyone experiences a sense of feeling empty at some time - it could be the result of a sense of loneliness, of sadness, of being abandoned, or even just simple fatigue or overwork in a meaningless job. Emotional eating is an attempt to fill that emptiness with food. Asking yourself if you're actually hungry or if this is something else often helps to clarify when the desire to eat is strictly emotional.

Taking a moment to mentally scan your body for other indicators can help. If you notice fatigue, tension, anxiety, these are indicators that maybe this is an emotional emptiness, not a hunger issue.

And of course, doing something else to fill the emptiness when it's an emotional issue is probably the most effective thing you can do to break the emotional eating habit.

There are lots of ways you can fill the emptiness, and each person will have different needs as well as different satisfiers that work for them. Being conscious of when it's an emotional "emptiness" and having a variety of ways of coping with that will make your healthy weight journey a lot more successful.

Make a list of the kinds of things that "fill your cup" - that is, fulfills your emotional needs so you don't have a desire to fill the emptiness with food or drink. Your list could include reading a good book, taking a walk on the beach, calling a good friend.

One of my friends has a book called **101 Kick Ass Things To Do Instead of Eating**. It includes tips for prevention as well as ideas to help you focus on what you are really needing - emotional connection, relaxation, etc.

You could add some of the ideas in the **101 Things** book to your list. Each person's list will be different. Keep your personalized list of 10 things handy for anytime you want an alternative to eating.

One of the keys to healthy eating and healthy weight is to recognize then your body is satisfied. Check in frequently while you're eating, especially in the early stages of changing your habits or patterns. Use your Hunger Scale and ask yourself where you are, on a scale from 1 to 10, in terms of feeling satisfied. If you are at a 4, slow down, you'll be at 5 pretty quickly. If you are at 8 or 9, then oops, you've gone overboard and next time you'll know to stop sooner.

Judy Wardell suggests that if you want to lose weight, keep your eating between 0-5. If you want to maintain your weight, then eat when you are between 3-7. If you want to gain weight, eat when you are between 5-10. Use the time before your meal - when you are giving gratitude for your meal - to check in with your Hunger Gauge.

Earlier we talked about eating 6 small meals a day instead of 3 larger "square" meals. The truth is, if you stop eating when you are satisfied, you will naturally need to eat more often since you are eating smaller meals.

The bottom line is to understand how *your* body works, and to work *with* it, not against it.

Food Research and How it Traps Us

The food industry in the United States has spent millions of dollars researching what it is that causes us to want to continue consuming food. This can be seen in the cereal foods that are advertised on TV. Most of them are sugary, and loaded with calories, hardly what you would call healthy.

The industry has learned that if they combined the right amount of sugar and salt, they can override our natural satiation trigger, thereby causing us to continue eating, even when we would normally be satisfied.

Most of us who have weight issues are no longer conscious of when our bodies are satisfied, and the food industry has made it harder. That means that in some ways we have "forgotten" where our true satisfaction level is, so we have to retrain ourselves.

When you think of your body as being the vehicle that takes you through life, you realize the true purpose of food is to fuel your internal engine so that you have the energy to take care of the things that are necessary in the physical world.

Where we get into problems is when we overfeed our engine (body). The extra fuel is not necessary, but our efficient engine continues to process it, and it ends up becoming additional padding or insulation that gets deposited on the inside and outside of our bodies. You'll avoid this problem when you keep your fuel gauge at 5 or below.

Whenever possible, stay away from processed foods. That can include soups and other canned goods. Get into the habit of reading labels to become familiar with the contents and levels of ingredients, especially sugars (including corn syrup and words ending in -ose, such as fructose, dextrose, sucrose, etc.) and salts (sodium). Remember that ingredients are listed in descending order of volume. If sugar is the first ingredient, you may want to reconsider whether you actually want to consume it at this time.

The real key here is to check in frequently with your body and assess where you are. It may seem difficult at first, especially if you've forgotten how to notice. Stick with it, though, and you'll be amazed at how much easier it becomes. This is one of the key strategies to helping control the portions you are eating.

You can help yourself relearn how to calibrate your hunger satisfaction by eating more slowly, only eating while sitting at the table, by focusing only on the food (no TV, no reading, etc.) and by taking the time to chew your food thoroughly.

Chewing is important for digestion, especially with vegetables. The digestive juices in your mouth are necessary to begin to break down the foods before they even get to your stomach. That in turn helps your body to better utilize the nutrients you are feeding it.

When you regularly eat smaller meals, your stomach gets used to recognizing when it's full (rather than overfull), and it gets easier and easier to know when to stop.

Managing Cravings

We all get cravings from time to time. The key here is to pay attention to the kind of craving you are having. Sometimes it's our body alerting us to a nutritional need. Other times it's a reaction to stress, tension, loneliness or some other emotional challenge.

Sometimes the solution is as simple as taking a walk, or drinking a glass of water. We'll discuss the importance of water in the next chapter.

The **kind** of food you are craving also gives you an idea of the source of your desire. If you find you are craving sweets or grains as a result of an emotional challenge, you may want to consider a quick and easy intervention.

The desire for comfort food - starches and carbohydrates like macaroni and cheese or baked beans - may signal a desire for connection with our past. For instance, being away from our family, or a desire to be close to our parents may trigger a desire to eat food similar to that we grew up with.

When it comes to weight issues, not dealing with emotional pain from our past is probably the main reason that those of us who are lucky enough to lose weigh in the first place can't seem to keep it off.

There are many ways to deal with emotional pain. Some people like talk therapy or other counseling techniques.

If you prefer to work by yourself, I've included some suggestions below and have provided links in the Resources section.

If you are willing to take a focused approach and make substantial changes, I highly recommend you consider meditation as a way to help you keep an emotional balance. Today there are many ways to do this - some of them very quick but still very effective.

People who meditate everyday are generally many times happier, healthier and live longer than those who don't. Even better, their sense of well-being is much higher than that of non-meditators.

For the past 7 years or so I have been using a product from Centerpointe called Holosync - sometimes referred to as the lazy man's way to meditate. It uses advanced audio technology to create the same brain waves as if you were engaging in Buddhist meditation. In the process, it can bring up emotional issues, which means that sometimes I find myself dealing with stuff that I wasn't expecting, but it's also expanded my ability to deal with emotional issues in general.

I started listening to the CDs back in 2004 when I had a high blood pressure scare. Luckily it turned out to be temporary, but in the meantime I made a ton of lifestyle changes, including watching the food I ate, adding specific supplements, increasing my exercise, and meditating using the Holosync CDs..

This is not a "quick fix", but something you may want to look into to see if it might suit your personal style.

I also use a process called the **Emotion Code** that helps people release emotional blocks so that their body can naturally heal itself. I was fortunate to get training directly from the originator, Dr. Bradley Nelson. It uses muscle testing, which in itself is a very useful testing device for discovering many things affecting the body, emotional balance and general health issues.

Muscle testing appears to tap into the unconscious and its regulation of the body, providing a physical response for issues that are below conscious recognition.

Another potential solution that is more immediate and does not require a lot of training is the **Emotional Freedom Technique** (EFT). It is simple and straightforward and uses acupressure points on the face and upper body to focus and release emotional issues. People have used it successfully for dealing with cravings for several years. I have seen it used very effectively to stop cravings for cigarettes. It's also used for pain control, release of emotional trauma, and other cravings.

In the Resources section is a link to a Kindle book that covers EFT as a way to deal with stress. I've also included a link to a video from Dr. Mercola - but he's not the originator of EFT nor even this particular video. You can find lots of videos available that explain and demonstrate EFT. Check them out on YouTube, or Google "EFT" to get more information. I am including Dr. Mercola's link because it is specifically focused on food cravings.

Next let's *examine the importance of water for your body...*

~Strategy 5~
Water - The Elixir of Life

Water is truly the miracle of life! Our bodies are mostly made up of water, and water covers the majority of the earth's surface. Drinking plenty of water keeps our bodies and our brains working properly. Lack of hydration can leave you feeling tired, confused and drained.

Water is a key component in any healthy weight loss program. The water in our bodies carries nutrients to our cells to nourish them. In turn, it carries away the toxins that are released into our blood stream as our body processes our fuel (food) and as the body starts to burn off the excess fat it's been storing.

Drinking plenty of water is essential, especially in the beginning of any weight loss plan. Since most of what you are losing when you begin a diet tends to be water, it's important for you to make sure you are replenishing what your body needs.

Many experts recommend drinking one-half your body weight in ounces every day. If you weigh 200 pounds, that means you should be drinking around 100 ounces of water every day. That's 12-1/2 glasses of water each day (8 ounces x 12.5 = 100 ounces).

While I personally consider this recommendation to be pretty accurate for me, it's also important to pay attention to the specifics of how your own body manages your water intake, and adjust as needed.

For instance, if you are physically active, or if you live in a warmer climate, you may need more water simply because you are losing moisture through sweating. If you are sedentary or in a cooler climate, you may not need as much. Each person is different, so adjust to suit your needs.

Sometimes we get what we think is a "hungry" feeling when we're really just thirsty. If you're not sure, drink a glass of water first. If you're hungry, you'll know soon enough. Some people even recommend you drink a glass of warm water about 20 to 30 minutes before every meal if you want to lose weight. The idea is that the water will give your stomach a sense of fullness and thus you'll eat less.

If you're feeling fatigued in the afternoon, instead of reaching for that sugary snack, consider a glass of water. Not only will you avoid the inevitable sugar crash after a temporary boost, you'll avoid those extra calories. And ultimately, you'll be giving your brain what it's really craving – water.

Fatigue may also be due to low potassium. You can counteract this fairly easily by having a half of a banana, or half cup of orange juice. When I used to fly a lot, I learned to mix my orange juice with sparkling water. The effervescent bubbles help push the potassium through the cell wall, relieving fatigue more quickly. Obviously, the better the source of your orange juice, the better it is for your health. Fresh orange juice is always preferable to concentrate, because then you are also getting the other nutrients.

Another secret that may help you maintain balance is to drink between 8 and 16 ounces of water (depending on your weight) as soon as you get out of bed, and before you eat. I have friends who swear by this practice. Again, your body has been fasting all night, and is probably dehydrated. Drinking water as soon as you awaken will help to re-hydrate your cells and further flush out any toxins accumulated during the night.

Simply put, water is an essential part of our lives. As we get older, the biggest problem we have to deal with is inflammation, which is the body's natural response to irritants. Chronic inflammation is a key factor in many serious illnesses, including heart disease and many cancers. We know that water helps to soothe, even on the inside of the body. In addition to healthy eating, drinking plenty of water is one of the most effective ways to remove the toxins that cause the inflammation.

It's also important to drink the purest water you can. It isn't necessary to buy bottled water, but if you have any concerns about the quality of your water, you can install a countertop purifier. Our water comes from a well, and when we moved into the house we installed a Multi-Pure under-the-counter water filtration system. We love it. Do your research and get something that works for you.

So now it's time to get moving ...

~Strategy 6~
Shake Your Booty

Exercise has often been touted as a key for losing weight. It certainly can help a sluggish metabolism, and is useful for maintaining weight loss. The problem is that many of us find the idea of "exercising" boring or a hassle.

Regardless of how we think about it, our bodies were designed for movement. Research has shown a direct link between physical activity and mental acuity. And over the years I've noticed how important movement is to strong mental functioning. When my father became wheelchair-bound and stopped walking, his mental faculties deteriorated rather dramatically.

In "olden days" we didn't need to worry about making sure we got "exercise". We were too busy bailing hay, planting the crops, stacking firewood, walking into town, etc. to worry about designing a workout at the gym. But today, with all of our modern conveniences, we have to be more mindful of getting enough physical exercise.

Certainly physical activity can improve our general wellbeing; reduce stress; strengthen muscles, bones and joints; elevate our mood; and improve our immune system..

In the past, many "exercise gurus" promoted aerobic exercise. Aerobic exercise raised the heart rate to a certain level and maintained it there for a long period of time. Aerobic exercises include activities such as jogging.

Many of the modern day "gurus" (including Dr. Mercola) are now advocating interval training. Interval training is the process of doing intense exercise for very short periods of time, followed by short periods of rest. For instance, doing wind sprints, or other activities that require short bursts of energy. The idea is that these short bursts of activity, followed by rest, and then repeated, are what help to provide optimum health.

If you think about it, this makes a lot of sense. Our bodies were designed to take care of things as the needs came up. For instance, at one moment we might have to run away from a large dog, or we might have to lift a large boulder and move it to a new location. But for the most part in our normal day-to-day activities, we were never designed to have sustained long periods of repetitive activity, such as running a marathon.

Maybe that's the reason I always liked baseball better than basketball or soccer. I played catcher so I was involved all the time, but it was intermittent activity, not sustained running. Even when I played 3rd base I didn't have to be "on" all the time.

There are many different ways to make sure your body gets the exercise it needs. Rather that telling you to do any specific kind of exercise, I encourage you to simply add movement into your life. That movement can be added in whatever manner makes sense to you, your current level of fitness, and your lifestyle.

It might take the form of walking around your neighborhood, using the stairs at work instead of the elevator, dancing to the music on the radio, doing yoga, taking hikes, walking on the beach, whatever gives you pleasure and gets you moving.

Personally I love to dance, and I've been known to turn up the radio loud so I can hear it where ever I'm working around the house. When the right music comes on, I often I stop what I'm doing and dance for 2 to 3 minutes and then go back to working again. I guess in some ways that's like interval training.

I also have several dance and exercise DVDs for times when I want a focused workout. Today you can get just about anything from Samba, to Tae Bo, to Yoga, Pilates and even more.

Some people adopt a dog as a way to force themselves to get exercise, knowing that the dog will need to get outside and walk everyday. I remember one time watching a young mother running after her very young kids - she was definitely getting enough exercise. In fact, I got exhausted just watching her!

Never underestimate the "built-in" opportunities around you.

Whatever you choose is up to you, but be sure to add movement into your life if it's missing, or increase it if you want more positive health benefits.

And of course, check with your physician if you have any questions about the appropriateness of the activity you are considering adding to your lifestyle.

And talking about lifestyles...

~Strategy 7~
The Power of Your Environment

The key to *maintaining* a healthy life is to create a lifestyle that supports you in being healthy and having the results you desire.

Your environment plays a huge role in your success. It includes your physical space, your family, community, all the things that you move through in your normal daily life. In many ways it defines the boundaries of your identity - both personally and professionally.

To create a supportive environment, sometimes you need to shift things around. For instance, if you are living in a rural area and you wanted to get a high powered executive job, you might need to move to a different location, or even to start your own business.

In regards to your health, you want to consider things that affect your ability to have the results you want - again, that's the physical, mental, emotional and spiritual. It can also include your job and the people you work with, or those you hang around with socially - your friends and associates. When you look at your environment, look at what's working now and what you may need to expand, exchange, let go of.

If your existing lifestyle is in conflict with what you want, you won't be able to maintain your program, no matter how strong your commitment nor how good your initial results.

Changing Habits

There are varying ideas about how long it takes to create a new habit - some people say 21 or 30 days, some say several months. Regardless, the new habit must be practiced over a period of time in order to become a natural, consistent, and unconscious aspect of your life.

Remember that a habit is simply a pattern that is focused on and repeated. It may be a pattern of thought or of activity. The key is that this pattern is repeated over and over again until it becomes integrated and treated as being something that is natural, normal and "real". In the psychological realm, this is called "conditioning".

If you want to get rid of an old habit, your best bet is to replace it with a new one. If you simply drop the old habit without replacing it, you'll have a vacuum, and vacuums tend to find something – anything - to fill themselves.

If you leave it up to the Universe to fill the vacuum, you are setting yourself up to be very unpleasantly surprised. Your mind is likely to find something very similar to what had been there before. This kind of defeats the purpose of eliminating a bad habit in the first place - you can actually end up just exchanging your original habit for something that's basically the same (or could be worse). This is why some people who quit smoking gain weight - they substitute putting *food* into their mouths instead of the *cigarette* that used to go there.

Even more important, if you want to be successful, you must **shift your identity** *first*, and then shift the habit. By shifting your identity to someone who does not have the problem, issue, etc., you automatically make it easier to let go of any habit tied to the old identity. Then, by replacing the old habit with something specific you would rather have, you are taking control of the process, and are much more likely to achieve and maintain the results you really want.

So first, decide what you want as a result of these changes you've set up for yourself. Ultimately it should be health related, and include easy weight maintenance. Short term, it could be about losing weight.

Next, we'll play a little mental game to help these changes seem real to you. This is an important part of shifting your identity.

Instead of maintaining the thought processes of yourself as you are now - the person who has the issue - you must see and experience yourself differently. You must **know** that you are capable of being this person and that you deserve to have the results you really want.

This is the piece that was always missing for me in regards to weight. But it really is the pivotal key to being successful, regardless of the change you want to make.

For example, I used to be a cigarette smoker. At one point I was going through three packs a day. Actually I was probably smoking a pack and a half because most of my cigarettes went out in the ashtray while I was working. Regardless, I decided I didn't want to be tied to that habit any longer.

I had tried several times previously to quit, but each time something stressful in my life brought me back to cigarettes. As a single person they were probably my most faithful companion, and at that point they'd been with me for 12 years.

This time, however, as I was going to bed one night, I simply threw away my partial pack and never lit another cigarette. That was 31 years ago.

I'm not saying I wasn't tempted. And I'm not saying the desire went away immediately. In fact for about five years I would sometimes wake up in a panic, thinking I had had a cigarette. I could even "smell" the smoke. But - I was only dreaming. It used to confuse me, but later I realized what a wonderful thing the mind is. My dreaming allowed me to have a cigarette without the bad effects! And without becoming habituated again.

I did something similar with caffeine - gave it up, cold turkey. But that time I had physical withdrawals that lasted for about three days. They were awful - in some ways worse than giving up cigarettes. But I persevered with that one, too. What

I found over time was that when I stopped jacking my system around with the stimulation of coffee, I had a much more sustained energy. I could go a lot longer than most other people because I wasn't relying upon artificial stimulation.

So, when the weight came back **one more time**, I finally decided to examine closely how I'd been able to suddenly turn off my cigarette and caffeine habits with relative ease and ultimate success. I also looked at what the conditions had been that allowed me to successfully **lose** the weight, even if I'd been less than successful in keeping it off.

What it Takes to Be Successful

There were several components to my success.

The first, and most important, was that NOW was the time. I knew that. There was no doubt in my mind. There was no "should", no "maybe", no "it would be a good idea". *I knew.* Deep inside I knew. No waffling. I wasn't beating myself up over having the issue. I just knew it was time to get rid of the weight once and for all. So, the first step was that it was time to make a change and I knew it. I was Ready.

Only *you* know if you're ready to do what it takes to have things be different. I'm guessing you are, or you're close to it - after all, you're reading this book.

A word of warning here, though: If you're *not* ready, just acknowledge that. Don't beat yourself up. Don't make yourself wrong. Do whatever you are currently doing, but do it whole-heartedly and with joy. If that means you're overeating - do it with loads of joy. Don't set yourself or your body up to make it worse by blaming yourself for your current behavior. That's craziness.

Remember, we all do the best we can with what we have at the moment. You'll know when you've had enough and you're ready to change your behavior. Casting blame never helped anyone. All it does is lead to opportunities to make excuses. You don't need excuses.

There is nothing inherently wrong with being a cigarette smoker or a coffee drinker (or with being fat). You get to choose. However, you need to be responsible for your choices. Remember, you are the "perfect you". Period. Own what you do.

Next I had to be willing to go through **whatever it took**. That was what I had faced when I tried all those crazy diets, and when I fasted. I knew it wouldn't be easy and I had to be willing to face all of it. I had to be willing to feel uncomfortable and I had to be willing to feel hungry. I had to be willing to stay the course. So, step two was my own Commitment.

I am reminded of the quote by W. H. Murray in *The Scottish Himalaya Expedition*, 1951:

> **Until one is committed, there is hesitancy, the chance to draw back, always ineffectiveness. Concerning all**

acts of initiative (and creation), there is one elementary truth the ignorance of which kills countless ideas and splendid plans: that the moment one definitely commits oneself, the providence moves too. A whole stream of events issues from the decision, raising in one's favor all manner of unforeseen incidents, meetings and material assistance, which no man could have dreamt would have come his way. I learned a deep respect for one of Goethe's couplets:

- *Whatever you can do or dream you can, begin it.*
- *Boldness has genius, power and magic in it!'*

Throughout my life I have found that every time I actually committed to something that was important to me, the process turned out to be a lot simpler and easier than I had feared. Putting it off and worrying about it had been a waste of time and energy.

Coincidentally, I was first exposed to this wonderful quote and concept in 1980, just before I gave up cigarettes for good.

In this case, the stream of events that issued from my decision was remembering I had written this great report on weight loss a few years ago. So I pulled it out and in the process of editing it, I realized there were still some pieces missing. That's when I decided to look more closely at those areas where I had been successful in the past.

Eureka!

That brought me to the most important step, **Shifting My Identity**. This is what had been missing from my weight journey. It was the essential key that made me successful where I had failed before. It's what insured that I would never go back to smoking: *I had shifted my identity from being a cigarette smoker to being a NON-smoker.*

This shift is essential. Once you are committed to change, there can be no going back. And that means you must **become** that to which you are **committed**.

For example, if you are a non-smoker, you would never seriously consider picking up a cigarette. It would be foreign to you - *not part of your identity*. And human beings will do almost anything to preserve our sense of who we are.

But, realistically, how many of us who have weight issues have made that shift? I certainly hadn't. While I felt great while I was losing weight, and even better once I was at my target, I still continued to feel like a fat person in a thin body. That was my very subtle self-sabotage.

I had continued to believe the things that had been said or implied to me. Things that other people had espoused as truth. I didn't question. I didn't reject. I didn't check in with myself. Or, when I did, it was to question myself, not them. At that point I had not yet developed, let alone completed, the exercises in this book so I had not yet reconnected with my own magnificence in any kind of permanent or meaningful way. I knew it was all there, but it was veiled by other people's opinions and beliefs.

Identifying this key element - *truly taking on the identity of the person you want to be* - was also essential to being successful in managing my weight. It seems so simple, yet elusive. It's a very subtle shift.

Most of us **want** to be different. We **hope** we can be different. But we continue to have doubts - our own, or those we've adopted from others.

When you **want** to be different, you are aware there **is** a difference. When you **want**, you habitually compare your **current** self to your **idealized** self, and that continues to point out the **lack** of being what you want to be - because you aren't there yet.

When you **hope** to be different, it's almost worse than **wanting** to be different. At least when you want to be different, sometimes you can forget that you are not yet there. When you **hope** to be different, you maintain a consistent mental comparison of both the current and future selves at the same time. That's why **hope** is usually such a wistful, but ineffective emotion.

The only way to successfully get around an issue is to go through it. Trying to avoid the truth, or make it something it isn't, simply won't work. If you have a weight problem, you have a weight problem, you're not big-boned or have a slow metabolism (even if those are contributing factors). If you're fat, you're fat. If you want to no longer be fat, you have to commit to becoming a not-fat person and then adopt the characteristics of a not-fat person. In other words, you must **shift your identity**.

Think about it: if you are a healthy person with a reasonable weight and body size - you would never consider typical "fat person" behaviors. You would eat to sustain your body, not overeat because you are trying to stuff some kind of feeling or upset. You wouldn't binge by eating a gallon of ice cream or a box of cookies. You wouldn't feel desperate for love or acceptance and take solace in food instead. You would eat what you wanted and leave the rest for another time. And you'd find something other than food to deal with your emotional issues.

And I'm not implying that all "naturally" thin people are happy, or that they don't engage in some kind of self-defeating behavior. It's just that most of them have a healthier relationship with food - they aren't consistently trying to make the food a substitute for something else they think they're lacking.

Every time I'd been successful in losing weight it was because of this shift - even if it was temporary.

Shifting Your Identity

We'll use this next process as a shortcut to facilitate the process of shifting your identity. Using only "normal" talk therapy type solutions, it could take you years to resolve these issues.

The time it takes for you to complete this process may be as short as 15 minutes or as long as 45. Set aside enough time to fully experience this process. Read through the following instructions or listen to it in the audio version. At the end, you may have already made the shift, or you may be several steps closer. As with the other processes in this book, you can come back to this again if you need a reminder.

Find a quiet place where you won't be disturbed.

Take a deep breath and close your eyes. As you let out your breath, allow yourself to begin to relax. Take another deep breath in and as you release it, also release any tension you may have noticed in your body.

For the next several minutes, we're going to play a game of "what if"... using the imaginary movie theatre in your mind.

First, think about your goals and dreams regarding health and weight. Think about the specifics - what you look like, how you move, what you feel like. Imagine that you have already accomplished what you set out to do.

I want you to imagine how great you feel as the "new you" - someone who is in control of your own body and life.

If you are someone who can form internal pictures, then picture in your mind's eye how you would look. Think about how you would feel and the kinds of things you would be doing.

Take the time to notice all the details.

If you're not someone who is comfortable making mental images, then just imagine what it would feel like if you already had those things that you really wanted and already were that person.

Imagine yourself there, in the picture, enjoying it all.

Imagine how good your body feels. How great it feels to be wearing clothes that are comfortable and stylish. See how good they look on you. Are you wearing a new style now? Notice how well your clothes flatter your figure and your image.

Using your internal images, notice the kind of life... friends... job... and home that the new successful you would have. Maybe not much has changed there, or maybe you decided to move and now you live somewhere you always wanted to live. Where ever you are, you are enjoying the company of friends, you are socializing with people who love you and are happy for you.

Ask yourself what kinds of habits this new you has incorporated that support the lifestyle you've chosen? Imagine yourself living the life that person would be living. See the interactions and imagine yourself actually experiencing them.

Think about the activities you would be engaged in. Are you playing sports? Going to the gym? Swimming? Tennis? Basketball? Jogging? Dancing? Weight lifting?

Imagine yourself doing those things the new you would be doing, and successfully responding to the old temptations from your new point of view. Imagine how you would feel in those situations, how simple and easy it is for you to make the right choices. Make your experience look, feel and sound as real as you can.

Make a mental note of how it feels for you to be in that situation, already having the results you most desire, being the person you want to be, and doing the things that are most important to you. Notice how the new identity feels.

At this point you now have all the clues you need in order to be that person and have that life.

Now take a moment, and wash the movie screen clean. Or imagine that the film has come to a close and it fades to black.

Think about that ideal person you want to become. The person who is comfortable in *their body. The person who is healthy and has a healthy relationship with food. The person who no longer needs to think about their weight - or about food - except as a way to fuel their body in a healthy manner.*

Notice the submodalities of that person. Where is the image located? Is it closer or farther away? Is it bright or dim? Clear or fuzzy? Color or Black & White? Still frame or movie? Are there particular feelings or physical sensations associated with the image of the person? Is there something you are saying to yourself? What else do you notice about it? Go ahead and write the submodalities down if that helps. Then finish the rest of this exercise.

*Next, think about who **you** are right at this moment. Imagine a picture of yourself on the screen. Notice the submodalities. Where is the image located? Is it closer or farther away? Bright or dim? Clear or fuzzy? Color or Black & White? Still frame or movie? Are there particular feelings or physical sensations associated with this image of you? Are you saying anything to yourself? What else do you notice about it?*

Pay attention to all of the differences.

Now that you know the submodalities for each image, begin to change each of the submodalities of the "current" you to the submodalities of the "new/ideal" you. Make sure that all of the differences go away. Make the "current" you exactly like the "ideal" you.

Take a moment and notice how you are feeling right now at this moment. Are you feeling comfortable in your new identity? Does it feel real to you? Have you noticed any shifts?

Now take the image you've been working on - the one where you changed the submodalities - and imagine that you move it into the same location as the "ideal" you.

Do you notice anything different? How does it feel? Did any of the submodalities shift back? If so, simply change them again to the "ideal" you. How are you feeling now?

Next, imagine you are merging the two images into one complete whole. How does that feel? Pay attention to the subtleties of how you feel now. Then bring that new image back to the location where the old current image used to reside. How does it feel there? Does it feel like it belongs?

Which location feels more comfortable for you? Which one feels "right" or looks "right"? Are there any subtle differences between how you feel in either location? Identify the one that feels best and most comfortable to you. It might also be a third, different location. Stay there.

When you are ready, you can open your eyes for the next part of the process.

Congratulations, this is the new you. This is your shift - whether partial or total. This is how you will interact with the world from now on. You haven't lost a thing - you've added appropriate behaviors to match your new goals. You still have all the resources you had before, plus the new ones you've identified that fit with the successful you.

What you've just done is to map the characteristics of the successful ideal-future-you onto your current self. That means you've re-coded your brain and shifted your identity. Most people notice a strong new sense of confidence and control as a result of this exercise.

This is similar to the "centered" feeling that athletes and martial artists access when they are preparing themselves for competition. In a similar way, from this point on, it will be easier for you to access the appropriate behaviors suited to someone who has a healthy relationship with food.

If you are not yet feeling comfortable as the "new you", you may want to go through the exercise again, looking specifically for differences between the two representations. There is likely a submodality that you missed. Once you identify and map that submodality across to your "current" image, you should be able to take on the new persona easily.

Staying Centered, Connected and Confident

And now your job is to continue to remind yourself and your mind that this new you is your dominant point of view. You will continue to do this until it becomes automatic for you, in other words, until it becomes a habit - your new habitual behavior - and you no longer need to consciously think about it.

For some people that will happen immediately. For others it may take more reinforcement before it becomes an unconscious part of who we are, directing our behaviors without conscious thought..

So, here's how you reinforce (or condition) it. Anytime you feel yourself slipping back into your old behaviors, or become uncertain about how to be in a new situation, simply do a quick check-in and compare the two identities (the "current" you and the "ideal" you). Focus on the "ideal" you, and shift submodalities that might need to be shifted so they match up again. Make sure you move your internal image to the location where you feel the strongest and most confident..

If you want, you can also set what's called a physical "anchor", that will help you recreate the experience if you want to access it as a resource to help with your resolve.

To do this, put yourself back into the experience of feeling strong, comfortable and confident. Intensify the feelings of being the successful you, and near the height of those feelings, create the anchor by rubbing your hands together, rubbing your arm, or making a clenched fist. Later, whenever you want to recreate that experience, the sense of being "centered", you can "fire" off the anchor by repeating the action that set it (for example by clenching your fist).

Some people have difficulty imagining themselves in the strong successful future position. If that's you, it's okay to start with someone else you know who has been successful in the way that you want to be. You will still do all the same steps, with that person's representation in the ideal-future-you position, and then you will map that person's characteristics onto your "current" self. This is called "modeling" - finding someone who has the results you want, and modeling their attitudes, behaviors, habits, etc., to get the same or similar results.

From here on out, you are a new person. You are operating in the world the way that ideal-future-you would be operating. You are not waiting for the changes in order to reap the rewards. You are being the change that allows the results to show up.

Be - Do - Have

Do you see the difference? Most people get it wrong - and in regards to weight, so did I for far too long. Most people think they need to DO certain things or HAVE certain things in order to make a change. Like, go on a diet, or buy a treadmill.

In reality, you must first BE the change, then everything else falls into place. When you ARE that new person, you will naturally DO the things that person does, and as a result, you will HAVE the body and health you want. And it will be relatively easy because you are simply doing the things that person naturally does. Any other way is a struggle because it requires willpower.

Gandhi's admonition to "Be the change you wish to see in the world," relates to our personal and internal world, too. It is much more difficult to force a change from the outside. It's disruptive and jarring - the way of revolutions. This is not to say it isn't one approach, just that it is often a difficult or painful one. And you often end up with unintended consequences.

When you make the change on the inside first, everything moves forward relatively easily from there. Everything you do, everything you are, operates in greater harmony. Even the answers to questions are more relevant and appropriate. It becomes the **source** of your choices, decisions and answers.

When I lost those 7 pounds on the cruise ship, I originally thought it was because of the effectiveness of the packaged food program I was on. With hindsight, I now realize it was because I had shifted into a state of "knowing" that whatever I was doing would work. And I was following the principles in these 10 strategies.

The program I was on included 5 small pre-packed meals that gave me just enough food to be satisfied, but never full. I was eating smaller, more frequent meals, and I was stopping when I was satisfied. Once a day the program called for a regular meal, watching for a balance of nutrients, and controlled portions.

While I was on the cruise, I basically ate what I wanted. But I didn't go crazy. For the most part I ate my 5 packaged meals, but sometimes it was only 3 or 4 because sometimes I ate meals provided by the cruise line, and sometimes we were out on a tour so I ate in a restaurant. And I ate desserts every day. They had beautiful desserts.

But I didn't eat the biggest, gooiest thing I could eat. Instead, I ate what appealed to me, which at the time was the plain cheesecake, sometimes with fresh fruit. And of the 8 days we were on the cruise, I had cheesecake for my afternoon snack at least 4 times and maybe more.

The other thing I did was to simply stop eating when I was satisfied. And because the dinners all included dessert, I made sure I stopped well before I was full. I wanted to enjoy the meal AND the delicious dessert. And sometimes I ate beyond a 5, but never beyond a 7.

So while at the time I thought my success was due to the program I was on, now I understand that it was due in larger part to the principles described in these 10 strategies. They simply work.

Reinforce your sense of this new you as often as you can. When you wake up in the morning, do a mental and physical check-in to make sure everything is in place. Make what ever adjustments are necessary to ensure all the submodalities are aligned properly. Do the same thing before you leave the house, or when you know you will be congregating with others, specially in settings where you might have felt ill at ease or less than worthy in the past.

As you sit down to a meal, make sure you are centered. Check your Hunger Scale. Give thanks for the food that will fuel your body. Focus on the process at hand and eat your meals when you are not distracted by other things. Check in often with your body and sense of balance. Stop when you are satisfied. That's basically it.

Create Supportive External Environments

Now that you have set up your own inner environment, the next thing you need to do is to make sure your external environment supports you in your healthy choices. You may want to make a list of anything you noticed while you were experiencing the last process that seemed to be important in helping you stay on track. Then begin immediately to set up these success systems in your life. Commit to making the changes that support you, and then start making them. Remember your commitment, and now own it.

This is the time to clean out your kitchen and refrigerator – get rid of the foods that don't support the new healthy you. Get rid of anything that could cause you to temporarily step away from the healthy choices the new you would make.

This could even include throwing out old clothes if you've been using your weight as an excuse to dress like a slob.

Begin to think about what you need to put in place that reflects the value (and the values) of the new you. From here on out, that IS you.

It's also essential to talk with the people closest and most important to you – your spouse or significant other, your children, your parents, and your friends. In fact, depending upon your relationships, it's probably best to let them know as soon as possible that you are making these changes.

Help them understand how important their support is. Let them know that you want their support, but not their judgment, and that you have a plan for what you are doing. The suggestions in this book are a non-traditional approach and the people around you may not understand why you aren't following a particular diet or plan they are familiar with.

Your friends and family may become resistant when they see you are making changes – they can become afraid that you'll leave them when you shift your habits and patterns from what they are used to with you. Sometimes they may even unconsciously sabotage your progress. You can help to allay their fears by letting them know that this is important to you and that their support is important, too. That you are counting on them because they are important to you.

Don't be surprised if some of your friends become uncomfortable with your progress. There are many reasons for this – perhaps they're afraid you'll leave them behind; perhaps they wish they could have the same results as you; perhaps your success reminds them of their own shortcomings.

If someone you care about is having strong negative reactions to your choices or your success, be patient with them if you can. Just as your choice of health is about you, their reactions are about them - not about you. Simply allowing them to be uncomfortable might be the most useful thing you can do. Sometimes, however, you may have to re-evaluate the relationship in light of the new you and your new lifestyle.

Choose to be with the people who will support you in being your best. Choose to put yourself into those settings where you can support yourself in maintaining your new choices and patterns. You are still growing, and positive growth is healthy.

10 Healthy Habits

To help create your supportive environment, identify ten healthy habits you can implement today and over the next couple of months. Make sure the habits are in alignment with your goals and desires.

Some suggestions include: doing yoga in the morning, sleeping in on Saturday morning, going fishing once a month with the guys, taking a walk every evening around the neighborhood. Find at least 10 healthy habits that you will enjoy and that support you in your new healthy lifestyle. These 10 things may be similar to the ones we looked at earlier regarding "filling your cup". They'll come in handy when you need to recharge your batteries or shift your current focus.

And finally, one of the most important things I learned from becoming a non-smoker is that you will continue to have temptations. Just don't obsess about them. For several months after I quit smoking, as I shifted my identity to that of being a non-smoker, I would sometimes have the thought, "I want a cigarette."

But I didn't obsess about it. And I didn't try to shove it away. You've heard the saying, "what you resist, persists"? At the time I hadn't yet heard that, but I knew that if I tried NOT to think about it, that I would just be making it worse. Telling your mind NOT to do something requires the mind to have to think about it FIRST before letting it go. That was not the result I wanted.

I discovered that if I simply **acknowledged** the thought, I could let it go. So when I got the thought, "I'd like to have a cigarette", I would mentally think, "yeah okay. I want a cigarette. So what. If I really want one, I can have one later." By acknowledging the thought and not denying it, it was just something that floated in and then out of my mind. Just another thought - not something I had to act on at that moment.

The other thing I did, at those times when the urge got strong, is that I substituted something else for the act of lighting up a cigarette.

Remember the 10 healthy habits? Well at the time I was a jogger, so if the desire for a cigarette became really strong, I would go out and run for a mile, or at least around the block. Later I learned that most smoking is a desire to relax - to breathe deeply. By running instead, I was satisfying one of the end results of smoking - deep breathing

If you find you are getting a strong desire for something that you know doesn't fit with your new persona, grab one of your healthy habits, something that fills your cup, or try something like a glass of water. You can also fix yourself something to eat that you really like, but is healthier.

One of the things I love is ice cream. Most ice cream has a huge amount of sugar, which I avoid for health reasons. Not only is sugar the cause of most obesity, it is at the root of most of the chronic health problems, especially in the U.S.

So, I've learned to stash some yogurt in the freezer that I can grab if I get that craving. Since I prefer plain Greek yogurt, instead of sugar I like to mix in some of that wonderful Saigon cinnamon - it gives enough flavor that I usually don't need any sugar. I also like to mix the yogurt with fresh strawberries or blueberries. If I do choose to add a sweetener, I use stevia or agave. Agave has a lower glycemic index, but it's still a sugar.

Does this mean I'll never eat ice cream? No. It means I won't keep it in the house. However, I do sometimes freeze those little sleeves of go-gurt, which can also be a good substitute. If I really want ice cream, I'll buy a cone or a cup while I'm out and about. That way I get to have exactly the flavor I want and when I eat it, I enjoy every bite!

Just remember, this is a journey. You'll be successful when you take it one step at a time ...

~Strategy 8~
Getting From Here
to There

It may sound trite, but you can only measure your progress if you're tracking it on a regular basis. If you've made the choice to become healthy and it includes releasing your extra fat, then you are probably not happy with what you look like right now, and the last thing you want is to be reminded of it.

Even if it seems painful right now, it's important to get an accurate idea of where you are starting from. I promise that once you start having success and dropping the pounds and inches, you won't remember what you looked or felt like when you started.

So, if you want to play full out, then grab a camera and a tape measure and log your starting point.

Take a full-on frontal shot and a side view of yourself. Measure your chest, waist, hips, thighs and upper arms. Weigh yourself on a good scale.

Remember these are simply data points - they don't mean anything by themselves. Write your data down in your journal or use the spreadsheet available in the Resource section at the end of this book. Record your thoughts about this journey to health you've chosen.

Some people like to write daily – what they've eaten, their measurements, and their thoughts about how they're doing. If it's important to you, I recommend you measure and write at least once a week.

If you are weighing yourself, try not to do it every day. Your weight will fluctuate several times every day, which could cause you to think that you weren't making progress. It will also change based upon your relative physical condition. Muscle weighs more than fat, so as you shift your body composition the pounds reflect something other than just excess fat. Set up a specific time and day of the week to check. You will get a more accurate picture if you only weigh yourself once a week.

You can even enter your weight or measurements into a spreadsheet like the one in the Resources section and create a graph if that inspires you. This is what I do - it encourages me to stay on track.

Be sure to celebrate your successes and record your milestones. Enter your new healthy habits and your healthy rewards. You may want to put everything into your journal, or put them up on a board. Add new pictures as the weight drops off. Write out your frustrations and challenges. Include how you moved back into alignment with being healthy any time you may have strayed.

As you progress along the path towards your goal, you will notice how different you feel – both physically and mentally. Writing out your thoughts can help you sort out the new feelings you may be having. It also provides a great reinforcement anytime you slip up and need to get back on track.

From time to time you are bound to move off course. This is normal and natural. It isn't inevitable, but still it can happen.

Just as your weight fluctuates on a daily basis, your nutritional needs will also fluctuate based on what is going on for you. Pay attention to any cravings that you may have.

The desire for sugar is generally an artificial craving as a result of already eating too many refined simple carbohydrates or processed foods. Anything other than a craving for sugar will generally mean that there's something your body needs and is attempting to acquire. Your body and your mind are designed to alert you to what you need in order to stay balanced.

If you find yourself in an occasional sense of overwhelm that results in you indulging in something that is less than healthy, notice what is happening for you. There's probably an emotional reason that triggered your response.

Rather than chastise yourself for backtracking, it's much more useful to ask what triggered the desire, what was going on emotionally and physically for you at the time that caused you to want to indulge or overeat. Sometimes it's as simple as stress, or just fatigue. These two things alone are significant reasons why so many people end up giving in to fast food and unhealthy snacks.

Lack of sleep can lead to many problems, not just fatigue during the day. Insufficient sleep at night increases your cortisol levels, which in turn adds to stress, which in itself can be a trigger to overeating or eating the kinds of foods that don't support your healthy body.

The important thing is to forgive yourself, eliminate the triggers when possible, and simply get back on track. If you can identify what was happening immediately before the trigger, you have a better chance to shift your reaction and short-circuit the trigger. Substitute one of the healthy habits instead.

Sometimes you may have to revisit the experience and set an anchor for healthy choices that you can fire off when you notice you are starting down the road to the trigger. After you set your anchor, reinforce it several times to keep it active. Then use it when you need.

If you find yourself sliding back down that slippery slope, go back to the earlier exercises. Reconnect with your source though the golden light, and then rediscover your ideal-future-self. Or simply use the anchor you created earlier. Talk to your support group. Read back through your journal. Just use whatever works.

Remember your commitment. It's your agreement with yourself. No one said it would be instant, but if you do these things (especially from the position of already having achieved your results), you'll keep moving forward, and that's the key.

If you want a physical reminder of your progress, keep one pair of pants (or one outfit) from your (heaviest) starting point. Periodically, or once you reach your goal, you may want to take a picture showing how big the clothes have become on you.

Once you reach your goal, buy a pair of pants that fit but are snug. Use these pants to help keep yourself on track – as soon as they begin to feel too tight, it's time to get back on your program!! And don't wait – do it right away!!

In the meantime, don't forget to celebrate ...

~Strategy 9~
Celebrate Your Progress!!

Just as you must replace old habits with new ones, it's important to create milestones along the way for any goal you set.

A milestone is a midlevel achievement, it's something that moves you closer to your actual goal, something that gives you a sense of accomplishment. It's not the ultimate goal, but it's significant because it shows progress and is measurable in real time. Depending upon your ultimate goal, you could have one or several milestones.

Life is about celebration, and celebration will help to keep you on track. As you approach your milestones, it helps to have a positive and healthy reward waiting for you.

Take the next 15 minutes and look back through your journal notes. Think about where you are, where you want to be, and what some logical milestones might be. Then brainstorm some appropriate rewards – almost anything other than food will do! Some ideas could be: a day at the spa, a massage, a pedicure, a new outfit, tickets to a sporting event, a new pair of hiking boots, anything that makes you feel special and rewarded for the extra effort you've put in!

Once you are in maintenance mode, you can even include food as a reward - for instance, in the form of going to a special restaurant. But, until you've mastered your new way of being, it's best to avoid all food-related rewards.

This is probably a good time to talk about alcohol on a weight program. Personally I think moderation in all things is a good idea. So I'm not opposed to alcohol. In fact, I drink a couple of times a week. Just remember that alcohol, like sugar, adds calories without nutritional value. So when you drink alcohol, you are using up nutritional calories and not getting any benefit. Remember, if you want to drink much, you can always increase your exercise or decrease your food intake as a trade-off.

As you look at your long term goals, set at least three milestones and assign a reward to each in addition to a special reward for reaching your final goal. Post your upcoming milestone on your refrigerator, your bathroom mirror, your computer monitor, any place where you will see it and be reminded that it's coming.

Now that you've identified the milestones, add them (and the rewards) to your journal. That way you can keep track of how you feel as you reach each milestone and enjoy each reward.

As you reach the milestones, think about what you have learned and what you have shifted. Think about who you have become, and what you could have told your earlier self that would have made the journey easier or more meaningful.

But also remember what Wayne Dyer said, "Your past is simply the path that brought you to where you are today." You don't need to return to the past. You don't need to worry about the past. It's over and done with, just as your old "fat" identity is over and done with. The past need never bother you again.

Life is a series of steps forward. Keep rewarding yourself and enjoy every step!

If you're smart about the way you create your milestone rewards, these can eventually become something that support you on a regular basis in maintaining your healthy lifestyle.

For instance, let's say you reward yourself for meeting a milestone by having a special massage. You could easily set up a biweekly or monthly massage as a reward for maintaining your weight.

In this way you are creating both a reward and a subsequent support system that works for you.

Now, let's look at some other support systems that may be useful ...

~Strategy 10~
Finding Your Personal Cheerleaders

Any good program requires support. A good support system is vital to the success of any new venture, even for your healthy weight loss journey. If you're lucky, your first level of support (after your own healthy choices and changes) will be your family or your significant other. If they can cheer you on, that's great!

As much as we might try to hide it, everyone around us knows when we are physically out of balance with extra weight. Sharing your goals with friends or with people who care about you can go a long way towards helping you stay on track.

There's also something about publicly declaring your goals. Most people seem to be more committed when they've publicly stated their intentions. This is part of our need to maintain and protect our sense of who we are. Encourage your friends to ask you how you're doing, and be prepared to report back with your results.

People also seem to be willing to do more for others than they are for themselves. Finding another person to share your journey with can be a huge motivator and a wonderful support system. It can help provide an accountability partner, as well as someone you are responsible for supporting.

Remember that your success can often motivate others to their own success. We are all connected in one way or another, and every success helps to support others in their own success, too, even it it's in a different area. When you can be a positive role model for others, your success also adds exponentially to your community.

Studies have shown that people who approach weight loss with an adequate support system are much more likely to successfully maintain their ideal weight over time. This is probably why programs like Weight Watchers, where people check in regularly with others, tend to work in helping people keep on track. This is even more reason to build support around yourself.

Ultimately your support groups include your friends and family, your neighbors, your doctors, your personal trainer if you have one, your work colleagues, any special organizations you belong to, and even your professional connections.

Even in my rural area, I have had several friends over the years who became walking partners. Sometimes they were close enough to just knock on my door in the morning, and sometimes we had to meet at the local park. Now that my husband is retired, we often take walks together. Where we used to spend time in the car on the way to work talking about specific things, now we do it on our walks.

If you don't already have some kind of health related support group in your community, you may be inspired to create your own group. Look around and find people that have similar values even if they don't have similar goals. These could be people at school, at work, in church groups, or in other organizations that you belong to. Or it could be a group that has no other interconnection except that you all want to support each other in your healthy weight journey.

Take a few minutes to list the organizations you already belong to. Identify how they might able to support you in this endeavor. Also list the key people in the organization you might hook up with. Consider who could support you, and identify specifically how.

Next make a list of the organizations or groups that might be helpful in supporting you in your health goals. These could be groups you'd like to join that have similar values to yours. Or they might include people who have the kind of physical, spiritual or financial success you'd like to have.

You might want to look for Zumba or Yoga groups, or a group that teaches you to meditate.

Finally make a list of the people you know that you can rely upon for support.

You may be surprised at who is willing to step up to support you or who might be available to play with you. Finding the right running partner or tennis partner might be simpler than you think.

Don't let your preconceived ideas stop you, you never know where the right partner might be hiding. And you won't find them unless you ask.

You may also want to consider hiring a trained Health Coach or Personal Trainer to help provide accountability and encouragement for your program.

A coach can work with you on your specific issues and can help educate as well as support you. Your coach will be a consultant who provides compassion, knowledge and professional assistance to help you maintain your commitment to health. A coach can help you course-correct when necessary, as well as provide long-term solutions to weight management challenges once you reach your goal.

Even if you don't choose a coach, find at least one other person that you know, like, and trust. Use this person as an accountability partner, someone you check in with on a regular basis.

If they can join you on your journey, all the better. It's incredibly useful to have someone who is working on the same health and wellness journey as you are. That way you can keep each other on track, brainstorm solutions when it's needed, and support each other when temptation strikes.

It's true that you can use your Health Coach or your Personal Trainer as an accountability partner, and sometimes that's the best thing to do when you're in the middle of a large goal. But most likely at some point you'll want to find someone you can personally relate to, especially as you transition into your new healthy lifestyle.

What To Do Next

My goal and intent for this book was to share the key concepts I discovered about what worked for me in attaining a healthy relationship with food.

Most of these strategies are based on common sense. But the insights that make them work are something that eluded me for many decades. I hope what you've learned here has given you some great ideas that you can implement in your own life.

Weight management, for those of us who have struggled with it, is a matter of remaining **conscious** about what and how we eat. Just as we learned behaviors that caused us to become fat, we can learn behaviors that can keep us thin and healthy.

There are a multitude of diets and programs that can help, and there really is no "one size fits all" solution. Some people do well with a strict diet, others with talk therapy, some with hypnosis. Some respond to behavioral modification and some naturally learn the process that works for them.

For me it's been a bit of all of the above. One program I was on was so successful for me that for a time I represented them as a Health Coach in addition to my Business and Career Coaching and hypnotherapy practice.

This was the program that required the use of pre-packaged food. That meant eventually I had to transition back to "normal" food. And that's where I fell off. My own coach at the time didn't prepare me as well as I'd hoped, and I didn't yet understand that I needed to shift my identity.

So as a "fat" person in a thin body, I did the only thing I understood at the time, I went back to my "normal" life, to my (fat) identity. Because nothing had fundamentally changed for me, even with my new understandings, my food and weight issues eventually caught up with me. Thank goodness that is now in my past.

If you adopt these strategies, there's no reason for you to have to restrict your diet to particular foods. In fact it's better to make sure you eat a variety of foods. That way you are less likely to become frustrated and go off a restrictive diet to binge on unhealthy foods. Of course it's best for you to have a healthy, balanced diet, but if you follow the ideas and techniques in these strategies, you can eat any of the foods you really want. You just don't get to eat huge quantities.

Remember to only eat when you are hungry, include a large quantity of fresh foods, and stop when you're satisfied - before you're full.

If you choose to use a diet program that includes specialized or pre-packaged food, I have some recommendations.

First, chose something that provides your body with the full nourishment it needs so that you can lose weight quickly without muscle loss.

Look for something that is affordable and within your budget - something that costs about the same as what you would spend on your food budget anyway. One of the problems with the low-carb and Atkins style diets is that the cost of buying lots of protein can increase your food budget - *unless you already eat a lot of protein or you eliminate other types of costly food purchases.*

Also look for something easy, something that requires very little preparation, and that accommodates a busy lifestyle. Otherwise you may find yourself falling off the program because it's too hard to maintain. And bottom line, we're here to be successful.

Any diet program you select should also help you identify and address the behaviors that contributed to the problem in the first place. You must be able to create a plan to implement the skills and habits that will help you successfully manage your weight and your new lifestyle.

The processes in this book are designed to do exactly that, regardless of whatever program you may choose to follow.

And finally, you will eventually transition back into the real world. That means if you have chosen a program that has restricted your food intake in any way - calorie or carbohydrate restriction, or pre-packaged food - you need a plan that will support you as you move back into the realm of temptation, and help you manage your new behaviors.

It's important to have your goals, desires, milestones, personal anchors, support system, and your environments in place.

This is also where a good coach or accountability partner can help you integrate everything successfully.

Again, if you've used the exercises in this book, all of this will be easier because it's a natural outgrowth of your new identity.

If you choose to simply modify your normal eating habits by adopting a new mindset as you shift your identity, then you are currently cementing the behaviors that will support you in your new lifestyle. You've already made the transition, and there's nothing to do but just keep it up.

Congratulations on your willingness to Master Your Inner Game. I wish you great success on your journey.

My Personal
Weight Loss Journey

Thank you for purchasing my book. It's my sincerest wish that what I've learned and shared here makes your journey easier. While the information itself is not earth shattering - after all it's not much different from what we're told by many health professionals - how you implement that information is what makes the difference between continuing to struggle and reaching your goals easily. Being in alignment with your body is the key to having success

Diets Don't Work

We've all heard this – and we know, deep down, that it's true. Weight Loss Diets don't work. They may be useful for a time, but eventually most of us fall off the wagon – in fact 85% of us will gain the weight back within two years unless we have some kind of behavioral support.

That's because anything that requires us to use willpower alone is bound to fail over time. The only lasting success comes when you permanently modify your relationship with food and that means modifying what and how you eat. And that also means having adequate support while you re-learn about your body and how to eat.

It's Really NOT Your Fault!

Many of us started the yo-yo diet journey in our teens and twenties. Some of us had no problems until we hit our 30s. And some of us discovered in our 40s that our bodies had changed so much that whatever we had used before simply no longer worked!!

Unfortunately we live in a society that values instant everything – from instant gratification to instant fast food to instant results! Any of these set us up for long-term failure.

There's no question the fast food industry has done more to obesify this country than anything else. And the glamour industry has done more to skew our self-images than anything else! We have both extremes – a population where 68% of us are overweight and 32% are obese – and a segment that is so concerned about extra pounds that they starve themselves into anorexia. Neither extreme is healthy physically or mentally. And both extremes have serious physical health consequences!

I Was In the Same Spot As You!

I have struggled with my weight ever since I hit puberty. At first it was only a few pounds – and because I was so physically active, it didn't hold me back very much. By the time I was a senior in high school, those few pounds turned into 20.

So I tried some variation of the Mayo Clinic Diet (remember that one – grapefruit and coffee and hardboiled egg breakfasts for two weeks). It seemed to work and I dropped 10 pounds. I still wasn't "optimum" but it was good enough for me.

Then I went off to college and out into the working world. Eventually, when I got pregnant with my daughter, my weight shot up 30 pounds. After she was born, I dropped 10, but then stayed there. After several months of again trying many different programs, a friend introduced me to the Atkins diet. Finally, it seemed I had found something that fit my personal body type and needs! After losing 30 or more pounds I was again feeling good about myself.

But low-to-no carbohydrates is difficult to maintain and even though I liked this diet a lot, eventually I again went back to my previous eating habits, unable to sustain the extremely low-carb lifestyle.

I Tried Some of the Strangest Diets!!

Over the years I have tried so many different diets I can't even remember most of them! There was the time I tried the South Beach Diet, the Grapefruit Diet, I even fasted for 6 weeks – drinking only water for the first week and then eating one grapefruit every 3-4 days. And eventually I would always go back to my most successful diet – the Atkins low carbohydrate diet.

The thing is, by then I was putting weight on pretty quickly – once even gaining 40 pounds in about 3 months. Nothing seemed to work but Atkins, but those results were short termed, too.

Then there was the time in my 30's when I became convinced that I was poisoning myself and I became afraid to eat. I would take a bite of food and it tasted strange, so I would spit it out. At the same time I started having difficulty swallowing so I kept a glass of water by me all the time and would take a sip every time I became afraid of not being able to swallow.

Needless to say, I lost a lot of weight during this time, and interestingly, after I got over whatever that poison fear was, I kept it off for two years – and I kept it off without even thinking about it. In fact, I figured I would never have a weight problem again because in that two year time I ate whatever I wanted, whenever I wanted, and had no issues with weight at all.

You know how the Universe steps in to remind you not to be so smug? Well you can guess what happened – at some point my "immunity" stopped and unfortunately the weight piled back on!

Eventually I went back on Atkins again and over a 9 month period I took off 65 lbs. This time it lasted about four years, but then we moved to the Redwoods, a beautiful but foggy place that does not encourage exercise, and the weight started creeping back on.

I Even Became A Vegetarian

During the mid-1990s I took Tony Robbins' Mastery University. During one of the programs I decided to try his recommendation to adopt a totally different way of eating – eating nothing but fruit until noon and vegetarian fare the rest of the day. Well, that was as far from Atkins as I could get and after 6 months and 40 more pounds I gave that one up for good!

I never really got used to so much sugar in my diet nor the lower protein and lack of dairy. I really missed the eggs and cheese – and believe me, there is no acceptable substitute for cheese.

Nothing Seemed to Work!
I Was So Frustrated...

Then an interesting thing happened...or rather, didn't happen. Suddenly, Atkins no longer worked for me. Oh, it would work for a couple days – long enough to get the water weight off, but then it would stop, and no matter what I did, I couldn't get it to kick in again!

Then my job became so stressful that I actually had to take two months off from work, and my weight went up again. I didn't realize it at the time, but stress causes increased cortisol – and that equals weight gain. So back on the yo-yo.

I tried counting calories. I tried portion control. I tried over the counter stuff from Costco and the pharmacies. I even tried some raw food & smoothie tricks. Nothing worked. I was getting desperate enough I even considered fasting again.

One of my friends elected bypass surgery and seemed to be doing very well with it. I toyed with that idea, but I don't like surgery and didn't like the finality of having my stomach stapled.

I kept remembering another friend who almost died because of an infection he got during the surgery and the friend who had such high hopes but only lost 20 pounds or the client who lost the weight after surgery and then put it right back on again.

Besides, I really wanted to be in charge of my life – not have some surgery limit it.

A Light At the End of the Tunnel?

When you are serious about your intent and ask in the right ways, the Universe brings opportunities to your door.

One day a friend shared a packaged-food diet with me. The program had more than 25 years of successful results. The reports I was getting from people on the program said not only were they losing 3-8 pounds a week, it was convenient and affordable, and they were having success..

I Couldn't Wait to Start!
Was This My Answer?

I got really excited and started right away. Although I didn't lose weight as fast as other people did, I eventually lost about 55 pounds over a 9 month period. I was ecstatic - finally something was working! But there were some problems – like my need for laxatives far more often than I liked – and making sure I carried extra food with me all the time because basically I could only eat what was packaged.

Then an interesting thing happened. I took advantage of a business apprenticeship opportunity that appeared to be exactly in the direction I was heading. Unfortunately, it turned out I was mistaken.

It took me four months to get myself untangled from the unscrupulous person I had trusted. And it took me another 12 months to recover all of the considerable money I had invested to become part of the apprenticeship program.

During that time I moved from confident and happy into feeling totally out of control – like I was walking on eggshells the entire time. And as a result, the weight came back on again.

Figuring Out What Works

That experience got me thinking about what had worked for me in the past. What I discovered that made a difference for is was that in order to be successful in a "diet" program, you absolutely MUST have three things:

- commitment to the program or plan
- guidance and support during and after
- a plan for transitioning back to the real world of food.

And, to be truly successful in regaining health and fitness, something much more fundamental is needed. You must shift your relationship with food, and ultimately, that means your relationship with yourSELF. Until you can do that, you will continue to struggle with weight, and be stuck on the dieting yo-yo.

I thought back to what it had taken for me to quit a 3-pack a day cigarette habit. I had been smoking for 12 years. I thought about how I'd quit "cold turkey" when I simply threw away my cigarettes and never smoked again. I thought about what I had gone through when I gave up caffeine.

Neither experience had been easy. I had gone through several days of severe headaches and nausea when I stopped drinking coffee, before everything evened out. And there were several years of waking up in a panic, thinking I had just smoked a cigarette, only to realize that it had simply been in my dreams.

The first time I had tried to stop smoking was as the result of a mutual agreement with my (then) boyfriend. The problem was, when we broke up, I went back to smoking. I had not chosen to stop for myself, it was part of an agreement with him. Now, there is nothing "wrong" with having a pact with someone - but the decision still MUST be made for yourself - not because someone else wants or expects you to do it.

It took me a few more attempts before I was successful. But from my current perspective of having shifted habits in the past, I now understood what worked and more importantly why it worked. So this time I decided to use the tools I'd learned and those I'd developed over the years to finally master my own food-weight-self relationship and stop the yo-yo.

If you want to be successful, one of the easiest ways is to model the mindset and behavior of someone who has the results you want. If you are unable to find someone else who has those results, then look for evidence in your own life of similar successes. Once you find something that is similar, it becomes possible to use that as a map for getting the results you want.

That's what I did. I used my successful results as an ex-smoker and as an ex-caffeine drinker.

If you're tired of trying diet after diet, if you're ready to make a healthy decision to regain the body you love, if you have a strong desire to look on the outside as beautiful as you are on the inside, using the exercises and following the guidelines in this book may be the answer for you.

If you want a safe and effective way to conquer this thing once and for all, if you want a program you can modify to meet your own body and lifestyle, if you want something that will be permanent and not just a fad, then this might be the road to success for you, too.

If you're thinking, "It can't be that easy!" you may be right. It takes a fundamental shift in your beliefs. If you're not willing to believe you're worthy of having the results, it will never happen.

It takes making a commitment and sticking to the plan. It takes your willingness to get right back on track again if you fall off. But isn't that true about anything in life? Or at least with anything worth having.

Maybe you're wondering how much of a hassle it might be? Well, if you want to focus your energies on things that empower you rather than having to count calories or carbs or fat, then give these strategies a try.

If you'd like someone to answer your questions, help you self correct as you learn what works for your body, provide ongoing support and cheer you on your way, then perhaps this is the time to find a Health Coach or other professional who will help you get and stay on track!

If you want to improve your chances for being successful, visit me at my website, **http://ABodyYouLove.com** and register for our newsletter. I don't send them very often, but I will keep you updated about my own progress, as well as send you occasional ideas and resources to make your progress easier

Recommended Resources

Websites

Dr. Mercola Nutrition Plan
http://www.mercola.com/nutritionplan/index.htm

Nutritional Typing - Dr. Mercola
http://nutritionaltyping.mercola.com/Login.aspx

Emotion Code - Dr. Bradley Nelson
http://www.drbradleynelson.com/

7 Minute Workout
http://bit.ly/VK9YD2
WARNING: This is a multi-level organization, but you can join just to use their videos and support system - that's what I do. They will give you customized videos to help you get the results you want. (This is an affiliate link.)

Books

101 Kick Ass Things to Do Instead of Eating
http://amzn.to/UwUxNO

Thin Within
http://amzn.to/ZpEZR0

How to Relieve Stress Using EFT
http://amzn.to/SlBNUy

EFT Video - http://youtu.be/L92oOPJlfyg
CenterPointe Meditation-
http://bit.ly/CtrPte

Other Resources By Katie Darden

Sign up at **http://ABodyYouLove.com/248-2/** to receive:

- Free Body Fat Calculator
- Weight Tracker (Spreadsheet)
- Information about how to purchase the audio version of the NLP/hypnosis processes

Katie's Books

Strategic Goal Planning Series (on Kindle)

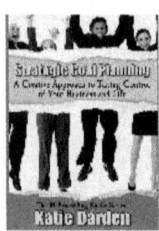

Determining Your Core Values:
  http://amzn.to/P1E12p
Creating Targeted Goals
  http://amzn.to/NW3aj7
Your Focused One Page Plan
  http://amzn.to/Ma3VGW

Collection of all 3 Books
  Kindle   -- http://amzn.to/YzgAmV
  Paperback -- http://amzn.to/WSkqIs

About the Author

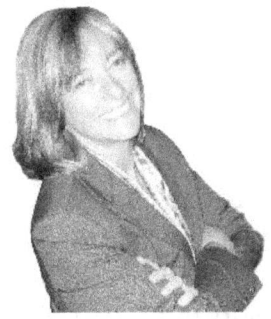

Katie Darden is a Business and Career coach, Trainer, Speaker and Internet Marketer with over 20 years experience in Human Resources, holding several different roles in government and private industry across a broad range of organizations, from small business start-up through City, County, State and Federal governments.

She's consulted for businesses such as Microsoft, Intel, Continental Airlines, Alcoa, Johnson and Johnson, Applied Materials, MCI, British Telecom, Glaxo, Hewlett Packard, Honda, Ontario Hydro (Canada), Syncrude Canada, US West, Department of Veteran's Affairs and several California State Agencies.

She is a 1997 graduate of *Coach U*, a founding member of *Coachville* and the *Graduate School of Coaching*, a certified Handwriting Expert, a registered and certified Hypnotherapist and Master Practitioner of Neuro Linguistic Programming (NLP).

She considers herself fortunate to live on the far Northern Redwood Coast of California and to spend the rainiest four months every year in San Felipe, Mexico, on the Sea of Cortez.

She enjoys creating environments and opportunities for people to discover and express their natural gifts and talents.

She congratulates you for being willing to keep looking for what works.

And she thanks you for buying her book.

www.ingramcontent.com/pod-product-compliance
Lightning Source LLC
Chambersburg PA
CBHW070704290526
45790CB00001B/441